ARTIFICIAL INTELLIGENCE IN MEDICINE

A Practical Guide for Clinicians

ARTIFICIAL INTELLIGENCE IN MEDICINE

A Practical Guide for Clinicians

Campion Quinn, MD

Rockville Medical, LLC, USA

World Scientific

NEW JERSEY · LONDON · SINGAPORE · BEIJING · SHANGHAI · HONG KONG · TAIPEI · CHENNAI · TOKYO

Published by

World Scientific Publishing Co. Pte. Ltd.

5 Toh Tuck Link, Singapore 596224

USA office: 27 Warren Street, Suite 401-402, Hackensack, NJ 07601

UK office: 57 Shelton Street, Covent Garden, London WC2H 9HE

Library of Congress Cataloging-in-Publication Data
Names: Quinn, Campion, author.
Title: Artificial intelligence in medicine : a practical guide for clinicians / Campion Quinn.
Description: Hackensack, New Jersey : World Scientific, [2024] |
   Includes bibliographical references and index.
Identifiers: LCCN 2023043573 | ISBN 9789811284106 (hardcover) |
   ISBN 9789811284564 (paperback) | ISBN 9789811284113 (ebook for institutions) |
   ISBN 9789811284120 (ebook for individuals)
Subjects: MESH: Artificial Intelligence | Medical Informatics Applications |
   User-Computer Interface
Classification: LCC R859.7.A78 | NLM W 26.55.A7 | DDC 610.285--dc23/eng/20231122
LC record available at https://lccn.loc.gov/2023043573

British Library Cataloguing-in-Publication Data
A catalogue record for this book is available from the British Library.

For any available supplementary material, please visit
https://www.worldscientific.com/worldscibooks/10.1142/13618#t=suppl

Desk Editor: Vanessa Quek ZhiQin

Typeset by Stallion Press
Email: enquiries@stallionpress.com

This book is dedicated to Anthony Calio, MD, a physician of unparalleled compassion, skill, and dedication to patient care. I'm proud to call him a friend.

Contents

Chapter 1

Artificial Intelligence in Medicine: Revolutionizing Healthcare

Artificial intelligence (AI) has emerged as a transformative force in the field of medicine, holding immense potential to revolutionize healthcare delivery and improve patient outcomes. In this introduction, we will explore artificial intelligence and its relevance in the medical field.

Objectives of this book

The objective of this book is to provide a review of the field of AI and its impact on medicine. The book aims to equip healthcare practitioners with the knowledge necessary to effectively utilize AI tools in their clinical practice. It covers fundamental concepts, practical applications, and ethical considerations associated with AI in medicine.

The target audience of the book is healthcare practitioners, particularly clinicians who may not have a background in computer science or artificial intelligence. The book is specifically designed to bridge the gap between AI and medicine, providing clinicians with the necessary knowledge and understanding of AI tools and their applications in clinical practice. It aims to empower healthcare practitioners to effectively leverage AI technologies to enhance patient care, improve diagnosis accuracy, personalize treatment plans, and utilize predictive analytics.

Recognizing the importance of preparing healthcare practitioners for the future of AI in medicine, the book addresses the ethical considerations and challenges associated with AI in healthcare, such as privacy concerns, potential biases, and limitations of machine learning algorithms. The book also provides strategies to deal with these limitations and offers guidance on the successful integration and adoption of AI technologies in clinical settings.

The definition of AI

The term "artificial intelligence" refers to the development of computer systems capable of performing tasks that typically require human-level intelligence.[1] Artificial Intelligence is a broadly encompassing term that includes but is not limited to, machine learning, deep learning, natural language processing, and computer vision. These systems are designed to simulate human cognitive processes such as learning, reasoning, and problem-solving. AI algorithms learn from large datasets, identify patterns, and make predictions or decisions based on the acquired knowledge. The goal of AI in medicine is to augment human capabilities, improve clinical decision-making, and enhance patient care outcomes.

A brief history of AI in medicine

The first use of AI in medicine dates back to the early 1970s when research produced MYCIN, an AI program that helped to identify blood infections treatments.[2] In 1979, the American Association for Artificial Intelligence was formed and ever since then, AI technology and machine learning have evolved to influence how healthcare is delivered. The early period of AI in medicine was important for digitizing data that later served as the foundation for future growth and utilization of artificial intelligence in medicine (AIM). Despite the lack of general interest during this time, AI pioneers continued to collaborate, and the first National Institutes of Health-sponsored AIM workshop was held at Rutgers University in 1975. The use of AI in medicine has since expanded and adapted to transform the healthcare industry by reducing expenditure, improving patient outcomes, and increasing overall efficiencies.

Today, the application of AI in medicine demonstrates remarkable achievements in various domains. One notable area is diagnostic imaging, where AI algorithms analyze medical images, such as radiologic, pathologic, and dermatologic images to assist in the detection and diagnosis of diseases. For example, AI algorithms have shown high accuracy in detecting diabetic retinopathy in digital photographs of the retinal fundus.[3] Another significant application is in dermatology, where AI models have achieved dermatologist-level performance in classifying skin cancer based on images.[4]

AI also plays a vital role in clinical decision support, helping healthcare professionals make informed treatment decisions by quickly providing access to relevant information and research. By analyzing vast amounts of medical data, AI algorithms can identify patterns and correlations that may not be readily apparent to human clinicians. For instance, researchers in UCSF used a deep learning AI model to accurately predict Alzheimer's Disease by analyzing patient's PET scans. This deep learning algorithm achieved an 82% specificity at 100% sensitivity, an average of 75.8 months prior to making the clinical diagosis.[5] This tool has demonstrated superior performance when compared to human experts, facilitating accurate and timely diagnosis and an opportunity for early therapeutic intervention.

The potential of AI extends beyond diagnosis and decision support. It holds promise in personalized medicine, tailoring treatments to individual patients based on their genetic profiles and specific disease characteristics. AI algorithms can analyze complex genetic and clinical data to predict treatment responses and optimize therapeutic interventions. Additionally, precision medicine could become easier to support with virtual AI assistance. AI models can learn and retain the preferences of its users. Therefore, AI has the potential to provide customized real-time recommendations to patients around the clock. Rather than having to repeat information with every new doctor or nurse, a healthcare system could offer healthcare workers around-the-clock access to an AI-powered virtual assistant that could answer questions based on the patient's medical history, preferences, and personal needs.

Moreover, AI technologies enable the analysis of vast amounts of electronic health record (EHR) data, unlocking valuable insights to improve population health management and identify trends in disease prevalence and treatment outcomes. AI and machine learning can play a key role in population health in the areas of data analysis, including predicting when a patient is at risk of ending up in the hospital, identifying patients who are at risk of developing chronic diseases, and identifying patients who are at risk of medication non-adherence. By leveraging AI, healthcare organizations can extract meaningful information from unstructured data, such as clinical notes, pathology reports, and medical literature, thereby facilitating evidence-based decision-making and enhancing research efforts.

The potential of AI in medicine

To illustrate the potential of AI in medicine, let's consider a few groundbreaking examples.

In one notable study published in the medical journal EYE in 2021,[6] researchers used an AI system in a community hospital that was capable of diagnosing diabetic retinopathy by analyzing retinal fundus photographs. The algorithm achieved an accuracy level comparable to human ophthalmologists, demonstrating the potential for widespread screening and early detection of this sight-threatening condition without the need for an ophthalmologist present.

A 2022 study from The Lancet, Combalia, Codella, and others, used AI algorithms to classify skin cancer based on dermoscopic images.[7] The study employed clinically realistic scenarios to simulate real-world conditions and assess the performance of AI systems in classifying skin cancer based on dermoscopic images. The models achieved dermatologist-level performance, highlighting their potential to assist in early detection and improve patient outcomes.

Furthermore, AI has shown promise in improving cardiac care. Cardiologist-level accuracy has been achieved in the detection and classification of arrhythmias using deep neural networks, enabling more efficient and accurate analysis of ambulatory electrocardiograms.[8]

As AI continues to advance in medicine, it is crucial to address ethical considerations and ensure responsible and equitable deployment. The World Health Organization (WHO) emphasizes the need to prioritize ethics and human rights in the design and use of AI in healthcare.[9] Striking a balance between the potential benefits and the ethical implications is crucial to maximize the positive impacts of AI in medicine.

Preparing healthcare practitioners for the future of AI in medicine

AI has the potential to enhance patient care by providing accurate and timely insights for diagnosis, treatment planning, and personalized medicine. Algorithms trained on vast amounts of medical data can assist healthcare practitioners in making more informed decisions, hence reducing errors and improving treatment outcomes.

An example of how an AI system can improve diagnoses and reduce errors is the CheXNeXt algorithm developed at Stanford University.[10] The researchers realized that while chest X-rays are the most common medical imaging test in the world, the interpretation of these tests is time-consuming and the number of X-rays that can be read is limited by a shortage of trained radiologists. For this reason, the researchers created a deep learning algorithm called CheXNeXt to evaluate chest X-rays. A retrospective comparison of the CheXNeXt algorithm to practicing radiologists showed that the deep learning algorithm performed at a similar level to radiologists in diagnosing 10 out of 14 types of diseases on chest radiographs. The results showed that CheXNeXt has the potential to expedite and democratize radiological evaluations, while improving accuracy and reducing physician burnout.

AI technologies can automate routine tasks, streamline workflows, and analyze large datasets much faster than humans. By automating administrative tasks, AI allows healthcare practitioners to focus more on direct patient care and spend their time and expertise where it is most needed. This can lead to improved efficiency, reduced workload, and increased productivity in healthcare settings. The healthcare industry is facing a shortage of skilled healthcare professionals,[11] and this gap is expected to widen in the future. AI can help fill this gap by augmenting the capabilities of healthcare practitioners, allowing them to handle larger patient volumes and provide better care to more individuals. AI tools, such as chatbots and virtual assistants, can provide initial assessments, triage patients, and offer basic medical advice, relieving some of the burden on healthcare professionals.

As AI is integrated into healthcare, it is essential for healthcare practitioners to understand the ethical implications and potential biases associated with AI algorithms. They need to be aware of the limitations and potential risks of relying solely on AI recommendations. By preparing healthcare practitioners for the future of AI, they can develop the skills and knowledge necessary to critically evaluate and interpret AI-generated insights, ensuring responsible and ethical use of AI in patient care.

AI is a rapidly evolving field — new advancements and research are emerging regularly. By preparing healthcare practitioners for the future of AI, they can engage in lifelong learning and stay up-to-date with the latest developments in AI technologies. This continuous professional development ensures that healthcare practitioners remain competent and proficient in utilizing AI tools and can adapt to the evolving healthcare landscape.

Ultimately, preparing healthcare practitioners for the future of AI in medicine is essential to leverage the benefits of AI technologies, improve patient care, enhance efficiency, address workforce challenges, navigate ethical considerations, and enable continuous professional development. By equipping healthcare practitioners with the necessary skills and knowledge, they can effectively integrate AI into their practice and utilize its potential for the betterment of healthcare delivery.

References

1. McCorduck P. (2004) In *Machines Who Think (2nd Edition)*, A K Peters Ltd.
2. Shortliffe EH, Buchanan BG. (1975) A model of inexact reasoning in medicine. *Mathematical Biosciences*, **23**(3–4), 351–379.
3. Raman R, Srinivasan S, Virmani S, Sivaprasad S, Rao C, Rajalakshmi R. (2019) Fundus photograph-based deep learning algorithms in detecting diabetic retinopathy. *Eye (London, England)*, **33**(1), 97–109.
4. Melarkode N, Srinivasan K, Qaisar SM, Plawiak P. (2023) AI-powered diagnosis of skin cancer: a contemporary review, open challenges and future research directions. *Cancers (Basel)*, **15**(4), 1183.
5. Ding Y, Sohn JH, Kawczynski MG, Trivedi H, Harnish R, Jenkins NW, Lituiev D, Copeland TP, Aboian MS, Mari Aparici C, Behr SC, Flavell RR, Huang SY, Zalocusky KA, Nardo L, Seo Y, Hawkins RA, Hernandez Pampaloni M, Hadley D, Franc BL. (2019) A deep learning model to predict

a diagnosis of Alzheimer disease by using 18F-FDG PET of the brain. *Radiology*, **290**(2), 456–464.

6. He J, Cao T, Xu F, *et al.* (2020) Artificial intelligence-based screening for diabetic retinopathy at community hospital. *Eye*, **34**, 572–576.

7. Combalia M, Codella N, *et al.* (2022) Validation of artificial intelligence prediction models for skin cancer diagnosis using dermoscopy images: the 2019 International Skin Imaging Collaboration Grand Challenge. *The Lancet Digital Health*, **4**(5), E330–E339.

8. Hannun AY, Rajpurkar P, Haghpanahi M, Tison GH, Bourn C, Turakhia MP, Ng AY. (2019) Cardiologist-level arrhythmia detection and classification in ambulatory electrocardiograms using a deep neural network. *Nature Medicine*, **25**(1), 65–69. Erratum in: *Nature Medicine*, **25**(3), 530.

9. World Health Organization. (2023) WHO calls for safe and ethical AI for health. https://www.who.int/news/item/16-05-2023-who-calls-for-safe-and-ethical-ai-for-health

10. Rajpurkar P, Irvin J, *et al.* (2018) Deep learning for chest radiograph diagnosis: a retrospective comparison of the CheXNeXt algorithm to practicing radiologists, *PLOS Medicine*, **15**(11), e1002686.

11. Association of American Medical College. (2021) The Complexities of Physician Supply and Demand: Projections From 2019 to 2034. AAMC Washington, D.C. https://www.aamc.org/media/54681/download

Chapter 2

What is Artificial Intelligence?

It is necessary for healthcare practitioners to understand the basics of artificial intelligence (AI) and its potential implications in healthcare. This chapter offers a non-technical overview of AI concepts, using explanations, and examples that are relevant to healthcare workers who may not have a background in computer science. To that end, this chapter will introduce several terms that are crucial to understand if one is interested in using AI to improve the practice of medicine. These terms include AI, machine learning, reinforcement learning, neural networks, natural language processing, predictive analytics, and computer vision.

Artificial intelligence key concepts and terms

The term "artificial intelligence" refers to the development of computer systems that can perform tasks typically requiring human intelligence. AI encompasses a range of technologies, including machine learning, deep learning, natural language processing, and computer vision. These systems simulate human cognitive processes, such as learning, reasoning, and problem-solving, enabling them to analyze data, identify patterns, and make decisions or predictions based on acquired knowledge.

To understand AI, healthcare professionals must understand some computer science terms that are used to describe AI systems. This is because knowing these terms will help healthcare professionals understand the systems and be better able to converse with their IT colleagues. Terms such as algorithm, machine learning, reinforcement learning, neural networks, natural language processing, predictive analytics, and computer vision, will be explained extensively throughout this chapter.

What is an algorithm?

One of the building blocks of AI is called an algorithm (Figure 1). In general terms, an algorithm is a set of rules to be followed when solving problems or performing specific tasks. An AI algorithm in the healthcare setting can be likened to a GPS navigation system. Just as a GPS system uses data to provide directions and make decisions about the best route to take, AI algorithms in healthcare use data to make decisions regarding patient care. Similar to how the GPS system considers various factors, such as traffic, road conditions, and distance to determine the best route to take, AI algorithms in healthcare consider various factors, such as patient history, symptoms, and test results to determine the best course of action for patient care. Like a GPS system, it can be adjusted to find different routes or locations, algorithms can also be adjusted to suit different healthcare contexts or patient populations.

These algorithms are more than just programming, they serve as specifications for various healthcare processes, such as calculations, data processing, automated reasoning, and decision-making. Just like in computer science, it is important to ensure that healthcare algorithms are correct and can accurately address the specific problem or task at hand. AI systems use algorithms and large amounts of data to learn, reason, and make decisions.

What is machine learning?

Machine learning is a subset of artificial intelligence. It is a computer system that can learn from data and adapt without explicit instructions. Machine learning systems improve their performance over time without requiring the user to change their programming. This is comparable to the training of a medical student. The medical student learns from examining and treating hundreds of patients and gradually becomes more accurate in diagnosing and treating conditions. In healthcare, machine learning algorithms can be used to analyze immense amounts of electronic health

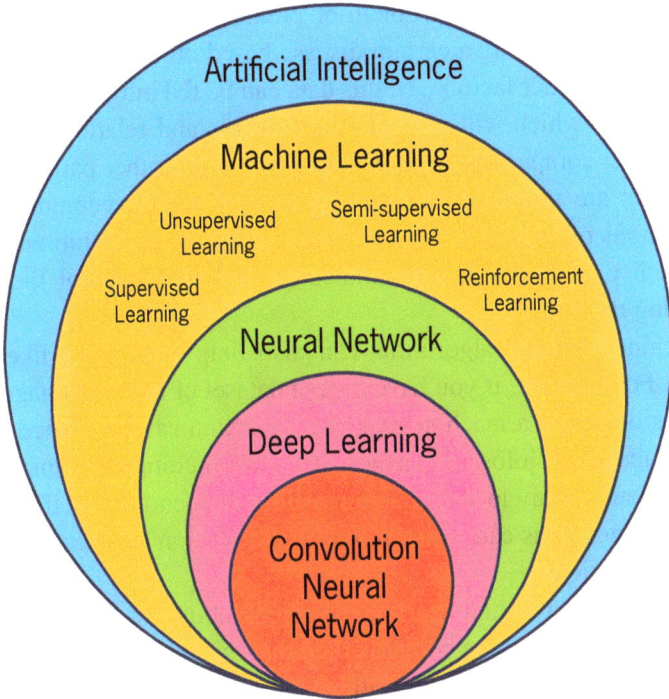

Figure 1. Artificial intelligence is an umbrella term for a group of technologies that include machine learning, neural networks, deep learning, and convolutional neural networks. Within the rubric of machine learning are the techniques of supervised learning, unsupervised learning, semi-supervised learning, and reinforcement learning.

record (EHR) data from millions of patients, thereby unlocking valuable insights to improve population health management and identify trends in disease prevalence and treatment outcomes.

Healthcare professionals encounter a vast amount of medical data every day of which they may absorb relatively little. Over the years, they can accumulate enough knowledge and clinical insight to become an effective clinician. Unlike people, machine learning algorithms can be fed millions of journal articles, reviews, reports, clinical images, and case studies within mere days and remember them all. They can analyze and summarize all the data to make decisions about medical care or predictions about the success of a type of therapy. The more data that they are fed, the more accurate those decisions and predictions become.

Take for example, the problem of predicting whether a patient is at high risk for developing a certain disease based on their medical history, lab results, and other factors. All this data can be fed into a machine learning algorithm, which will examine the patterns and relationships within the data, then compare the patient data with all the other patient medical records that are stored in its memory, as well as the recommendations from millions of journal articles. Subsequently, the algorithm will generate a prediction or a risk score indicating the likelihood of the patient developing the disease.

Machine learning algorithms can also help with tasks like image analysis. For instance, if you have a large dataset of medical images, such as X-rays or MRIs, a machine learning algorithm can be trained on millions of labeled radiological images. It can then compare them to a particular patient's x-ray to detect abnormalities or identify specific features in those images. This can assist in the early detection of diseases or guide treatment decisions.

The power of machine learning lies in its ability to find patterns and make predictions based on complex data that may be difficult for humans to analyze manually. These algorithms can uncover subtle relationships and trends that might not be immediately apparent to human observers. Here are a few examples:

Disease diagnosis

Machine learning algorithms have shown promise in diagnosing diseases based on various data sources. For instance, in dermatology, a machine learning model trained on a large dataset of skin images can detect subtle patterns or features indicative of skin cancer or other dermatological conditions that might be overlooked by human observers.[1]

Disease progression

By analyzing longitudinal patient data, machine learning algorithms can identify patterns in disease progression. For example, in the case of neurodegenerative disorders like Alzheimer's disease, machine learning models can detect subtle changes in brain imaging data over time, allowing for early identification and prediction of disease progression that might not be readily apparent to clinicians.[2]

Treatment response

Machine learning algorithms can analyze patient data, including clinical records, genetic information, and treatment outcomes to identify patterns related to treatment response. By considering a wide range of factors, such as genetic markers, demographics, and comorbidities, these algorithms can predict which patients are likely to respond well to specific treatments, enabling personalized medicine approaches.

Prognosis and survival analysis

Machine learning models can integrate various patient data, such as clinical variables, laboratory results, and imaging findings to predict patient outcomes and survival rates.[3] These models can identify subtle risk factors or combinations of factors that contribute to disease progression or survival probabilities, providing clinicians with valuable information for treatment planning and patient counseling.

Researchers developed a machine learning model to predict survival in patients with glioblastoma, an aggressive type of brain cancer.[4] The model was trained on a dataset of over 500 glioblastoma patients, which included variables such as age, tumor location, surgery extent, gene expression profiles, and MRI radiomic features. The model was able to predict each patient's risk of 6-month mortality with over 90% accuracy. It identified associations between specific imaging features, gene expression patterns, and survival that were not apparent with traditional statistical methods. For instance, the model found that certain texture patterns on MRI of the tumor as well as an elevated expression of hypoxia-related genes were indicative of higher mortality risk. This model was able to provide clinicians with accurate and personalized survival estimates for newly diagnosed patients. By revealing these prognostic factors, it could assist doctors in selecting more or less aggressive treatment plans and counseling patients more accurately on their prognosis. Machine learning tools like this have potential to significantly improve outcome prediction in glioblastoma and other cancers.

Adverse event detection

Machine learning algorithms can analyze large-scale healthcare data, including EHRs and adverse event reporting systems to detect patterns associated with adverse events or medication side effects.[5] It is important to note that while machine learning algorithms can provide valuable insights and enhance decision-making, they should always be used as tools to complement and support the expertise of healthcare professionals. Collaboration between AI systems and healthcare professionals can lead to improved patient care, more accurate diagnoses, and better treatment outcomes.

Machine learning can be understood by considering a scenario in which the objective is to predict the likelihood of a specific disease in a patient. To achieve this, the machine learning algorithm can be provided with the relevant patient data, including the patient's medical history, lab results, genetic information, and other factors. The algorithm then analyzes the data, identifies patterns, and compares this patient's patterns to the patterns of other patients whose diagnoses is already known. From this analysis, the machine learning system can make accurate predictions about the patient's diagnosis and possible disease course.

In another illustration, consider a scenario where the focus is on predicting the risk of cardiovascular disease (CVD) in patients. The algorithm examines the data of multiple patients, including their medical history, lab results, lifestyle factors, and genetic markers related to CVD. Through its analysis, the algorithm discovers specific combinations of risk factors that are strongly associated with the development of CVD. These risk factors could include a family history of CVD, high cholesterol levels, smoking habits, and a sedentary lifestyle. By recognizing these patterns, the algorithm can generate a risk score indicating the likelihood of an individual patient developing CVD. This risk score serves as a valuable tool for clinicians in implementing preventive measures or closely monitoring high-risk individuals. For instance, if the algorithm determines that a patient has an elevated risk score, healthcare providers can recommend lifestyle modifications, prescribe appropriate medications, or suggest regular check-ups to manage the patient's risk effectively.

This approach utilizes machine learning to leverage the power of data analysis and pattern recognition to make predictions and assist healthcare professionals in providing personalized care based on an individual's risk profile. By continuously refining its predictions through learning from new cases, the algorithm can improve its accuracy over time and contribute to better healthcare outcomes.

However, machine learning algorithms are not without their disadvantages.[6] For example, deep learning algorithms are very sensitive to noise in their data input. Even a small error or noise in a labeled data point can have a significant impact on the entire model. As deep learning algorithms learn iteratively, errors can propagate and affect subsequent steps, potentially leading to inaccurate predictions or classifications. This sensitivity to noise highlights the importance of ensuring the accuracy and quality of labeled data used in training deep learning models.

Another disadvantage of deep learning algorithms in the healthcare context is their complexity, and that complexity has a cost. Deep learning algorithms are more sophisticated than traditional supervised or unsupervised algorithms, requiring more computational resources and specialized hardware. The training process of deep learning models often involves large-scale datasets and complex software architectures, which can be computationally intensive and time-consuming. Healthcare providers may need to invest in powerful hardware and infrastructure to support the training and deployment of deep learning models effectively. For example, in healthcare applications, deep learning algorithms may be used to analyze medical images, such as X-rays or MRIs, for disease detection or diagnosis. However, the noise sensitivity of deep learning algorithms means that even a small error in the labeled data can affect the accuracy of disease classification. Similarly, the complexity of deep learning algorithms requires healthcare providers to have robust computational resources to process and analyze large volumes of medical imaging data efficiently.

Healthcare providers need to be aware of these disadvantages and consider them when implementing deep learning solutions. Steps should be taken to ensure the quality and accuracy of labeled data used for training deep learning models. Additionally, healthcare organizations should carefully evaluate their computational infrastructure to ensure it can handle the demands of deep learning algorithms effectively. Despite these challenges, deep learning holds great potential in transforming healthcare by enabling more accurate disease diagnosis, personalized treatment plans, and improved patient outcomes.

While deep learning can help to make more accurate diagnoses, these algorithms are not meant to replace health professionals. Instead, they ought to act as tools that can assist healthcare providers in making more informed decisions. They can help to prioritize patients, identify high-risk individuals, suggest treatment plans, or provide decision support based on the available evidence. By utilizing machine learning algorithms, clinicians can tap into the potential of vast amounts of medical data to gain valuable insights and enhance diagnostic accuracy.

Types of machine learning

Several types of machine learning algorithms can be used in healthcare. Some of the most common types of machine learning include supervised learning, unsupervised learning, semi-supervised learning, and reinforcement learning.

Supervised learning

In supervised learning, the algorithm is trained on labeled data to make predictions or decisions based on the data inputs. This type of machine learning is used for classification and regression problems, such as identifying pathologies in X-rays or MRI scans. These types of scans generate a large amount of visual data. Supervised learning algorithms are trained using labeled medical images, where the labels indicate the presence or absence of specific conditions or diseases. The algorithm learns to recognize patterns and features in the images that are indicative of certain diseases or conditions. Once trained, the algorithm can analyze new, unlabeled medical images and make predictions about the presence or likelihood of specific diseases or conditions. This type of machine learning algorithm can assist doctors in making quicker and more accurate diagnoses based on the analysis of medical images.

Unsupervised learning

Unlike supervised learning algorithms, unsupervised learning algorithms can identify hidden patterns and groupings within unlabeled healthcare data. This can be valuable for medical professionals since labeling vast amounts of patient data can be infeasible. Two common unsupervised techniques are clustering and association analysis.

Clustering looks for similarities between items in a dataset. Then, it divides data points into distinct clusters based on those similarities. For example, researchers used clustering on genetic data from thousands of patients to identify cancer subtypes that responded differently to treatments. This revealed distinct molecular profiles within a single cancer diagnosis.

Association analysis identifies relationships between variables based on co-occurrence patterns. It has been used to detect adverse drug reactions by finding associations between medications and symptoms documented in electronic health records. Another example is using association mining to discover comorbidities, which are conditions that co-occur more often than by chance. By discovering subgroups and associations, unsupervised learning provides insights from complex unlabeled data. It has great potential to improve clinical decision-making and knowledge discovery as healthcare systems amass vast amounts of data. However, human clinical expertise is still required to interpret the patterns identified and determine their practical significance.

One example of the use of unsupervised machine learning in healthcare is a 2021 Hong Kong study, where researchers were able to identify clinical phenotypes across the disease spectrum in patients with COVID-19.[7] The study used an unsupervised machine learning clustering approach to better understand the different clinical phenotypes across the disease spectrum in patients with COVID-19. The algorithm identified four clusters of differing clinical phenotypes based on their admission data. They found that 87% of the patients that died from COVID-19 were in a single phenotypic cluster. The clinical patterns captured in this cluster analysis were validated in other temporally distinct cohorts in 2021. The study demonstrated the usefulness of unsupervised machine learning techniques with the potential to uncover latent clinical phenotypes in patients with COVID-19.

Semi-supervised learning

In semi-supervised learning, the algorithm is trained on a combination of labeled and unlabeled data. This type of machine learning is used when labeled data is scarce or expensive to obtain. An example of the use of semi-supervised machine learning in healthcare is the development of predictive models for patient outcomes. In this case, the algorithm is trained on a combination of labeled and unlabeled data to predict patient outcomes based on their medical history and other factors. The algorithm can be used to identify patients who are at higher risk for adverse outcomes, allowing healthcare providers to intervene early and improve patient outcomes.

Consider this hypothetical example of how semi-supervised learning can be helpful in a clinical context: A researcher is developing an AI system to detect pneumonia on chest X-rays. They have a small, labeled dataset of 300 X-rays annotated by radiologists as either pneumonia positive or negative. However, the researcher also has access to a large trove of 100,000 unlabeled x-ray images. To develop an accurate pneumonia screening tool, more labeled training data is needed. However, having radiologists manually review and label 100,000 X-rays would be incredibly time-consuming and expensive. This is where semi-supervised learning can help. The researcher can use both the small, labeled dataset and the abundant unlabeled images to train the model. Techniques like self-training, pseudo-labeling, and generative models allow semi-supervised algorithms to take advantage of unlabeled data. The model learns to recognize visual patterns of pneumonia from the labeled data. Then, when analyzing the unlabeled images, the model progressively improves by using its predictions on these images as extra training signals. This enables the model to bootstrap its performance beyond the original 300 labeled examples. With semi-supervised learning, the researcher is able to create a highly accurate pneumonia screening tool while minimizing the need for costly manual annotation. This demonstrates the value of semi-supervised techniques for developing AI systems in healthcare when labeled data is limited.

Consider a real world example. A study published in medRxiv by researchers at the University of Toronto used semi-supervised machine learning to develop phenotyping algorithms for electronic health records (EHRs).[8] The researchers used a combination of labeled and unlabeled data to train the algorithm to identify patients with specific medical conditions. The algorithm was trained on a large amount of unlabeled data (i.e., unreviewed medical records) and a small amount of labeled data. The algorithm was then used to identify patients with specific medical conditions based on their EHR data. The study demonstrated that semi-supervised machine learning can be an effective method for developing phenotyping algorithms for EHRs.

In practice, the choice between these learning paradigms depends on the specific use case, the data available, and the resources at hand. Semi-supervised learning is often a good choice when there is a limited amount of labeled data but a large amount of unlabeled data. In terms of computational efficiency, semi-supervised learning can be less efficient than unsupervised learning since it often involves more complex models and training procedures that need to handle both labeled and unlabeled data. However, it can be more computationally efficient than fully supervised learning when the latter requires a larger labeled dataset for similar performance.

Reinforcement learning

Reinforcement learning is a machine learning technique that focuses on training AI systems to make a sequence of decisions to maximize rewards or minimize penalties. It is inspired by how humans and animals learn through trial and error. This type of machine learning is used for decision-making problems, such as optimizing treatment plans for patients. In reinforcement learning, an AI agent interacts with an environment and learns by receiving feedback in the form of rewards or punishments based on its actions. The goal of the AI agent is to discover the best actions to take in different situations in order to maximize the overall cumulative reward. Through repeated interactions with the environment, the AI agent learns which actions lead to positive outcomes and which ones should be avoided.

To illustrate this concept, consider a relevant example for clinicians, whereby an AI system is being trained to develop personalized treatment plans for cancer patients. The AI agent interacts with the patient's medical history, genetic data, and response to prior treatments. Based on this information, the AI agent tries different treatment options and receives feedback on the patient's response and outcomes. If a treatment leads to positive results, such as tumor shrinkage or improved quality of life, the AI agent receives a reward. If, however, a treatment has negative side effects or worsens the patient's condition, the AI agent receives a penalty. In AI, rewards and penalties serve as feedback to guide the system towards actions that best meet its goals, a process at the core of reinforcement learning. This feedback mechanism is also applied in other machine learning approaches to refine parameters and enhance outcomes. Over time, the AI assimilates this feedback, crafting strategies that are increasingly effective and personalized for individual patients. Reinforcement learning has been successfully applied in various areas relevant to healthcare professionals. In robotic surgery, for example, reinforcement learning algorithms can train robotic systems to perform surgical procedures with precision and adaptability.[9] The AI agent learns from previous surgical cases, incorporating feedback from expert surgeons, and improves its performance over time. This can potentially enhance surgical outcomes and patient safety. Another application of reinforcement learning in healthcare is optimizing resource allocation in hospitals. AI systems can learn to make decisions about bed allocation, staff scheduling, and resource utilization based on patient demand and available resources.[10] By continuously learning and adapting to changing conditions, reinforcement learning algorithms can help hospitals operate more efficiently and improve patient flow and care coordination.

Understanding reinforcement learning can help healthcare professionals appreciate how AI systems can learn from experience and dynamically adapt their decision-making processes. This has the potential to enhance personalized medicine, treatment planning, surgical procedures, and resource management in healthcare, ultimately leading to improved patient outcomes and more efficient healthcare delivery.

Neural networks

Neural networks are a powerful subset of machine learning algorithms that draw inspiration from the structure and functioning of the human brain. They are designed to mimic the way our brain processes information and recognizes patterns. Neural networks consist of interconnected nodes called called neurons that are organized into layers.

Each neuron in a neural network receives input signals, which can represent various features or characteristics of the data being analyzed. These inputs are then processed by the neuron through a mathematical function, which applies weights to the inputs to determine their significance. The weighted inputs are summed up and passed through an activation function to produce an output. This output serves as the input for the next layer of neurons in the network, and this process is repeated until the final layer produces the desired output.

Neural networks excel in tasks such as pattern recognition, classification, and regression analysis. For example, in medical imaging, neural networks can be trained to analyze images and identify specific features or anomalies that may indicate the presence of a disease or condition. This can aid clinicians in making accurate diagnoses from radiological images such as X-rays, MRIs, or CT scans.

Deep neural networks

A deep neural network (DNN) is an advanced artificial neural network architecture used for machine learning tasks like image recognition, natural language processing, and medical diagnosis. DNNs contain substantially more hidden layers than standard shallow neural networks, which enables them to learn highly complex relationships within data.

In a neural network, each layer is composed of interconnected nodes that process input data. The input layer receives the raw data, while multiple hidden layers detect patterns and extract features. Each hidden layer recognizes increasingly abstract representations of the data. With many hidden layers, DNNs can identify intricate hierarchies and relationships that shallow networks cannot. The final output layer generates classifications or predictions. The depth of DNNs provides immense modeling power. As data propagates through the many layers, each layer interprets the data in a more sophisticated way. The chained layers thus build up an intricate understanding of the data. This deep learning enables DNNs to take in raw data like images or text and perform accurate computer vision or language tasks. The multitude of layers empowers DNNs to capture subtle nuances and data complexities beyond the capability of traditional neural networks. DNNs excel at discovering latent structures within messy, high-dimensional data.

The ability of DNNs to learn hierarchical representations of data is particularly advantageous in solving complex problems. By leveraging the depth and complexity of the network, DNNs can automatically learn and discover intricate patterns and relationships in the data. This makes them well-suited for tasks such as image and speech recognition, natural language processing, and even autonomous decision-making. Compared to traditional neural networks, DNNs have the potential to achieve higher levels of accuracy and performance in many AI tasks. However, training and optimizing deep neural networks can be more challenging due to the increased number of layers and parameters involved. DNNs require large amounts of labeled training data and significant computational resources to train effectively. Advanced techniques such as regularization, dropout, and batch normalization are often employed to prevent overfitting and improve the generalization ability of DNNs.

In medical applications, DNNs have shown promising results. For example, in dermatology, deep learning models can analyze images of skin lesions and provide predictions on whether the lesion is benign or malignant, assisting dermatologists in making informed decisions for skin cancer diagnosis. Similarly, in the field of genomics, deep learning algorithms can analyze DNA sequences to predict the likelihood of genetic disorders or personalize treatment options based on an individual's genetic profile. By leveraging the capabilities of neural networks, clinicians can benefit from advanced technologies that help them interpret complex medical data more accurately and efficiently. Neural networks enable automated analysis and interpretation of medical images, text-based medical records, and genetic data, providing valuable insights that support clinical decision-making and improve patient care.

Natural language processing (NLP)

NLP is a branch of artificial intelligence that focuses on enabling computers to understand, interpret, and generate human language. It allows machines to interact with humans in a more natural and meaningful way, just like how healthcare professionals communicate with patients. NLP enables computers to understand the context, semantics, and nuances of human language, helping to extract valuable insights from textual data and facilitating communication between humans and machines. To put it simply, NLP enables computers to "read" and "understand" text, similar to the way a clinician reads and understands medical records, research papers, or patient notes. Here are some examples of how NLP is being used in medicine today:

Clinical documentation

NLP algorithms can analyze clinical notes and other textual documentation to extract important information such as diagnoses, symptoms, medications, and treatment plans. This can help clinicians save time and improve accuracy in creating comprehensive patient records.

Voice assistants

Voice assistants like Amazon's Alexa or Apple's Siri utilize NLP to understand spoken commands and provide relevant information or perform tasks. In healthcare settings, voice assistants can help healthcare professionals access patient data, schedule appointments, or retrieve medical information hands-free, thereby improving workflow efficiency.

Information retrieval

NLP algorithms can search through massive amounts of medical literature and research papers to extract relevant information based on specific queries or topics. This assists clinicians in staying up-to-date with the latest medical advancements and evidence-based practices.

Clinical decision support

NLP can be used to analyze patient data, including medical histories, lab results, and imaging reports to provide real-time clinical decision support. For instance, NLP algorithms can flag potential drug interactions or alert healthcare profesionals to relevant clinical guidelines, helping them make well-informed decisions at the point of care.

Sentiment analysis

NLP techniques can analyze patient feedback, reviews, and social media data to gauge public sentiment and opinion on healthcare services, medications, or treatment approaches. This information can be used to improve patient satisfaction, identify areas of improvement, and enhance the overall patient experience.

Patient monitoring

NLP algorithms can process and analyze unstructured patient data from sources like patient-generated health data, social media posts, or online forums to identify potential health risks, monitor patient sentiment, or detect early signs of disease outbreaks or adverse events. These are just a few examples of how NLP is being applied in medicine. NLP algorithms use techniques like text classification, named entity recognition, sentiment analysis, and language modeling to make sense of textual data. By enabling computers to understand and process human language, NLP can assist clinicians in extracting valuable insights from medical texts, improving communication, and supporting clinical decision-making processes.

It is important to note that while NLP has made significant advancements, it still faces challenges in accurately understanding complex medical jargon, interpreting context-specific information, and maintaining patient privacy and data security. Nevertheless, NLP holds great promise in transforming how healthcare professionals interact with technology and harnessing the power of textual information for improved patient care and healthcare outcomes.

Predictive analytics

Predictive analytics is a powerful aspect of artificial intelligence that leverages historical data to make informed predictions about future patient outcomes. It is like having a crystal ball that can forecast how the health of a patient may progress based on their medical history, genetic information, and response to treatments. This technology enables clinicians to identify individuals who are at a higher risk of developing specific conditions or experiencing adverse events, empowering them to take proactive measures and develop personalized care plans.

To understand predictive analytics, consider the scenario of a clinician treating a patient with diabetes. By analyzing the patient's medical history, including previous lab results, treatment regimens, lifestyle factors, and genetic markers, predictive analytics algorithms can identify patterns and relationships. These algorithms can then generate predictions about the patient's future health outcomes, such as the likelihood of developing complications like cardiovascular disease or kidney problems. This information helps the healthcare professional tailor the treatment plan to mitigate these risks and optimize the patient's long-term health. Another example where predictive analytics can be valuable is in the field of oncology. By analyzing enormous amounts of patient data, including tumor characteristics, genomic information, treatment protocols, and outcomes, predictive analytics algorithms can identify patterns and associations. This enables clinicians to predict the response to specific cancer treatments, anticipate potential side effects, and customize treatment plans based on the individual's unique characteristics. For instance, predictive analytics can help determine which patients are more likely to benefit from certain chemotherapy regimens or targeted therapies, hence improving treatment efficacy and minimizing unnecessary treatments.

Predictive analytics can also play a crucial role in population health management. By analyzing large-scale health data from a diverse group of individuals, including electronic health records, claims data, and social determinants of health, predictive analytics algorithms can identify trends and risk factors associated with certain diseases. This information allows clinicians to identify subpopulations at higher risk of developing conditions like cardiovascular disease, diabetes, or mental health disorders. With this knowledge, healthcare providers can develop targeted interventions, implement preventive measures, and allocate resources more efficiently to promote better health outcomes for the population.

It is important to note that while predictive analytics has immense potential, there are challenges to consider. The quality and accuracy of data, data privacy and security, and the interpretability of complex algorithms are areas that require careful attention. Additionally, predictive analytics is not intended to replace a healthcare professional's expertise but rather augment their clinical decision-making process by providing valuable insights and predictions. Predictive analytics in AI enable clinicians to utilize historical data to forecast patient outcomes and identify individuals at higher risk of developing specific conditions or experiencing adverse events. By leveraging these predictions, healthcare professionals can proactively intervene, develop personalized care plans, and optimize patient outcomes. Whether it be managing chronic diseases, predicting treatment responses in oncology, or improving population health, predictive analytics holds tremendous potential for revolutionizing healthcare and enabling more precise and individualized patient care.

Computer vision

Computer vision is an area of AI that empowers computers to comprehend and interpret visual information from images or videos, just like humans do with their eyes. It involves developing algorithms and models that allow computers to extract important features, identify objects, recognize patterns, and understand the content of visual data. Think of computer vision as a virtual set of eyes for the computer. It enables the computer to "see" and analyze images and videos in a way that is like how a clinican examines a patient. Instead of relying solely on text-based information, computer vision helps the computer understand and make sense of visual data.

In healthcare, computer vision plays a crucial role in various applications. For instance, consider medical image analysis. Just as a healthcare professional examines medical images like X-rays or MRI scans to diagnose and understand the patient's condition, computer vision algorithms can be trained to analyze these images automatically. These algorithms can detect abnormalities, highlight regions of interest, and assist healthcare professionals in making accurate and timely diagnoses. Another example relevant to healthcare professionals is the use of computer vision in facial recognition systems. Just as humans can recognize faces and distinguish between different individuals, computer vision algorithms can be employed to automatically identify and verify individuals based on their facial features. This technology can have applications in patient identification, access control to secure medical records, and monitoring patient movement within a hospital setting.

By understanding computer vision, clinicians can grasp how AI algorithms can process visual information, like their own visual perception, and make informed decisions based on what they "see." This has vast potential in healthcare, ranging from medical image analysis to patient identification, and can support healthcare professionals in making accurate diagnoses, enhancing patient care, and improving overall healthcare outcomes.

Conclusion

This chapter has discussed the immense potential that AI holds to transform medical practice and improve patient care. From assisting in diagnostics and personalized medicine to revolutionizing drug discovery and enabling remote healthcare, AI offers valuable tools and insights for healthcare professionals. AI can be seen as a trusted ally, aiding clinicians in diagnosis, treatment planning, and improving patient outcomes. However, medical practitioners need to stay informed, engage in ongoing education, and collaborate with AI technologies responsibly to maximize the benefits while upholding patient safety, privacy, and ethical standards.

References

1. Das K, Cockerell CJ, Patil A, Pietkiewicz P, Giulini M, Grabbe S, Goldust M. (2021) Machine learning and its application in skin cancer. *International Journal of Environmental Research and Public Health*, **18**(24), 13409.
2. Kavitha C, Mani V, Srividhya SR, Khalaf OI, Tavera Romero CA. (2022) Early-stage Alzheimer's disease prediction using machine learning models. *Front Public Health*, **10**, 853294.
3. Yoon JH, Pinsky MR, Clermont G. (2022) Artificial intelligence in critical care medicine. *Critical Care*, **26**(1), 75.
4. Chang P, Grinband J, Weinberg B, Bardis M, Khy M, Cadena G, Su M, Cha S, Filippi C, Bota D, Baldi P, Poisson L, Jain R, Chow D. (2018) Deep-learning convolutional neural networks accurately classify genetic mutations in gliomas. *American Journal of Neuroradiology*, **39**(7), 1201–1207.
5. Choudhury A, Asan O. (2020) Role of artificial intelligence in patient safety outcomes: systematic literature review. *JMIR Medical Informatics*, **8**(7), e18599.
6. Babic B, Cohen IG, Evgeniou T, *et al.* (2021) When machine learning goes off the rails: a guide to managing the risks. *Harvard Business Review*, **99**(1), 76–84.
7. Lau KY, Ng KS, Kwok KW, Tsia KK, Sin CF, Lam CW, Vardhanabhuti V. (2022) An unsupervised machine learning clustering and prediction of differential clinical phenotypes of COVID-19 patients based on blood tests — a Hong Kong population study. *Frontiers in Medicine*, **8**, 764934.
8. Yang S, Varghese P, Stephenson E, Tu K, Gronsbell J. (2023) Machine learning approaches for electronic health records phenotyping: a methodical review. *Journal of the American Medical Informatics Association*, **30**(2), 367–381.

9. Ma R, Vanstrum EB, Lee R, Chen J, Hung AJ. (2020) Machine learning in the optimization of robotics in the operative field. *Current Opinion in Urology*, **30**(6), 808–816.

10. Feng D, Zhiyao T, *et al.* (2021) Data-driven hospital personnel scheduling optimization through patients prediction. *CCF Transactions on Pervasive Computing and Interaction*, **3**(3), 40–56.

Chapter 3

An Overview of Data Collection, Preprocessing, and Feature Extraction in AI

Introduction

In the field of healthcare, data plays a critical role in enabling the capabilities of artificial intelligence (AI) systems. Data serves as the lifeblood of AI, providing the raw material that fuels its intelligence and powers its capabilities. Just like a huge library filled with books, data can be seen as a treasure trove of information waiting to be explored by AI systems. Each piece of datum holds valuable insights, stories, and facts that contribute to the AI system's understanding of healthcare.

Data takes various forms, ranging from structured data like organized rows and columns in spreadsheets to unstructured data like text documents, images, and audio recordings. These diverse types of data hold their significance and contribute to the AI system's knowledge base. For example, medical images can be analyzed by AI systems to detect diseases, text data can be processed to extract clinical insights, and patient records can be analyzed to predict health outcomes. Data on its own is a raw representation of facts or instructions that lack context or meaning. It requires interpretation and processing to transform it into useful information. Data is processed by computers using algorithms and logical operations to produce new data or meaningful output based on input data.

In a healthcare context, data refers to information related to health conditions, reproductive outcomes, causes of death, and quality of life for individuals or populations. It encompasses various types of data collected and used when individuals interact with healthcare systems. This includes clinical metrics, such as records of services received, conditions treated, and clinical outcomes, as well as environmental, socioeconomic, and behavioral information pertinent to health and wellness. Data can be created by users, software applications, or hardware devices connected to a computer system. It can be stored and recorded in various forms, such as magnetic, optical, electronic, or mechanical media. Data is transmitted between systems or devices as digital, electrical, or optical signals. The use of data is essential in medical AI systems. Data serves as the foundation for training and developing AI models that can assist healthcare professionals in various aspects of patient care. The availability of large and diverse datasets, such as population health datasets or medical claims and billing data, enables AI algorithms to learn patterns, make predictions, and provide valuable insights to support clinical decision-making.

A primary motivation for integrating data into AI systems is to improve the precision and efficiency of medical diagnoses and treatment plans. By analyzing large amounts of medical data, including electronic health records (EHRs), medical images, genomic data, and scientific literature, AI algorithms can identify patterns and associations that may not be readily apparent to healthcare professionals. These algorithms can help in the early detection of diseases, risk assessment, and personalized treatment recommendations based on individual patient characteristics. Additionally, data is essential for training AI algorithms to interpret medical images accurately. Medical imaging techniques such as X-rays, MRIs, and CT scans generate large volumes of data that can be utilized to train AI models to detect abnormalities, classify diseases, and assist radiologists in their interpretations. This can improve the efficiency of image analysis, reduce the chances of misdiagnosis, and aid in identifying critical findings that may be overlooked. Moreover, data plays a crucial role in enhancing the operational efficiency of healthcare systems. By analyzing data related to patient flow, staffing, scheduling, and supply chain management, AI systems can help hospitals optimize their operations and improve the quality of care. These insights enable healthcare providers to allocate resources effectively, streamline processes, and enhance patient access to healthcare services.

It is important to ensure the quality and diversity of data used in AI systems because the biases and limitations in the data can impact the performance and fairness of AI algorithms. This can potentially lead to disparities in healthcare delivery. Therefore, efforts are being made to address these challenges and promote the use of representative and inclusive datasets to train AI models that provide accurate and equitable support to healthcare professionals. Before all this data can be used, however, it goes through a series of steps that include data collection, preprocessing, and feature extraction.

Data collection

Data collection is the first step where scientists gather all the necessary medical information from different sources before being processed in an AI system. These sources include:

- Electronic Health Records (EHRs): EHRs contain comprehensive patient health information, including medical history, diagnoses, treatments, laboratory results, and medications. These records are collected and stored by healthcare providers and hospitals during patient visits.
- Medical imaging: Medical imaging data such as X-rays, MRIs, CT scans, and ultrasounds provide visual representations of the patient's anatomy and can help diagnose and monitor diseases. Images are captured using specialized equipment and stored in digital formats.
- Wearable Devices and Internet of Things (IoT) Devices: With the increasing popularity of wearable devices, such as fitness trackers and smartwatches, physiological data like heart rate, activity levels, and sleep patterns can be collected continuously. IoT devices, such as remote monitoring systems and sensors, also contribute to the collection of patient-generated data outside of healthcare facilities.

- Clinical trials and research studies: Research studies and clinical trials collect data from participants to investigate the effectiveness and safety of new treatments, interventions, or medical devices. These studies generate valuable data that can be used for AI analysis and to improve patient care.
- Health apps and patient portals: Mobile health applications and patient portals allow patients to record and track their health information, such as symptoms, vital signs, medication adherence, and lifestyle habits. These apps enable individuals to actively participate in managing their health and contribute to the collection of personal health data.
- Social media and online communities: Social media platforms and online communities provide a wealth of health-related information and patient experiences. Analyzing these unstructured data sources can uncover insights and trends that contribute to AI-driven healthcare improvements.

Once the data sources are identified, the collection of medical data involves various methods, such as:

- Data entry: Healthcare professionals enter patient information into electronic systems manually or through predefined templates during patient encounters.
- Data extraction: Data extraction techniques involve retrieving relevant information from structured and unstructured sources, including EHRs, medical reports, scientific literature, and research databases. Natural Language Processing (NLP) and text mining methods are often used for data extraction.
- Data integration: Healthcare data from different sources, such as EHRs, medical images, and genetic data, may need to be combined and integrated for a comprehensive view of the patient's health. Integration techniques ensure that data from multiple modalities can be analyzed together effectively.
- Data privacy and security: Strict protocols and regulations are in place to protect patient privacy and ensure the security of medical data during collection, storage, and transmission. These include measures like anonymization, encryption, access controls, and compliance with data protection laws like HIPAA.

Data preprocessing

After collecting the data, it needs to be "cleaned up" before it can be used. That is, the data needs to undergo preprocessing to assure its quality, consistency, and usability. The following are some of the steps involved in preprocessing:

- Data quality: Preprocessing helps to ensure data quality by identifying and handling issues like missing values, outliers, noise, and inconsistencies in the dataset. These issues can impact the accuracy and reliability of AI models. Noise in data refers to irrelevant or meaningless information that is present within a dataset. In the context of data analysis and machine learning, noise can cause significant problems, leading to inaccuracies in analysis and predictive modeling. By cleaning and refining the data, preprocessing improves the reliability of the input, ensuring that the data used for analysis is trustworthy and representative. For example, if a dataset contains missing values for a patient's blood pressure measurements, preprocessing techniques can be used to handle these missing values and avoid inaccurate analysis or predictions.
- Data standardization: Preprocessing involves standardizing the data to a common scale or format. This step is important when dealing with features that have different units, ranges, or distributions. Standardization brings the data into a consistent range, preventing certain features from dominating the model's learning process due to their larger values. For instance, if a dataset includes patient weight measurements in pounds and heights in centimeters, standardization can transform these variables into a common metric, making them comparable and ensuring that no single feature dominates the analysis based on its magnitude.

Handling categorical data

Preprocessing techniques address the challenge of dealing with categorical variables in AI models. Many real-world datasets contain categorical variables, such as disease types or medication names, which need to be transformed into numerical representations. A common approach to handling categorical data is called "one-hot encoding." This is a technique used to represent categorical data in a format that can be easily processed by computer algorithms. In medical practice, we often encounter different categories or options for variables such as diagnoses, medications, or patient characteristics. One-hot encoding helps convert these categorical variables into a numerical format that can be used for analysis and predictions.

As an example, consider a hospital that wants to build a model to predict patients' risk of readmission based on data from EHRs. One feature in the data is admitting diagnosis, such as pneumonia, heart failure, sepsis, etc. Representing the raw diagnosis labels directly could cause the model to incorrectly infer a medical hierarchy. Instead, the data scientists utilize the one-hot encode diagnosis feature to avoid this issue. Each unique diagnosis value becomes its own binary feature column. To illustrate this, a patient admitted for pneumonia would have the vector [1, 0, 0, 0, 0] where 1 is the index for pneumonia, while a patient with heart failure admission would be [0, 1, 0, 0, 0]. With diagnosis codes encoded this way, the model cannot make false assumptions about ranking or hierarchy. Pneumonia is not treated as "less than" heart failure. This prevents biases and improves the model's ability to accurately assess each patient's readmission risk independently of diagnosis code semantics. One-hot encoding is crucial for handling categorical features like diagnoses or demographics when modeling clinical data. It ensures the machine learning model interprets the categories correctly.

As another example, consider a scenario involving patient data related to diabetes diagnosis, and the following categorical data for diabetes diagnosis is obtained:

Diagnosis: ['Type 1', 'Type 2', 'Gestational', 'Prediabetes', 'No diabetes']

In one-hot encoding, each category in the diagnosis field is represented as a separate binary feature. Therefore, the one-hot encoding of this data would look as follows:

- 'Type 1':   [1, 0, 0, 0, 0]
- 'Type 2':   [0, 1, 0, 0, 0]

- 'Gestational': [0, 0, 1, 0, 0]
- 'Prediabetes': [0, 0, 0, 1, 0]
- 'No diabetes': [0, 0, 0, 0, 1]

In this way, each category is transformed into a unique binary vector. This binary value is like a "flag" that indicates the presence or absence of a specific category. It is worth mentioning that this transformation expands the dimensionality of the dataset, which can be a consideration depending on the size and complexity of the data.

The purpose of one-hot encoding is to prevent the introduction of any numerical relationships or order between the categories. It allows us to treat each category as a separate and independent variable when analyzing the data. This is important because assigning arbitrary numerical values to categories could lead to incorrect interpretations or biases in the analysis. By using one-hot encoding, we can transform categorical data into a numerical format that computers can understand and analyze. It enables us to leverage the power of computer algorithms to gain insights from complex data and make more informed decisions in healthcare. One-hot encoding has applications in various areas of healthcare and research. For example, in medical research, it can be used to analyze the effectiveness of different treatment options or to predict patient outcomes based on various characteristics. It can also be helpful in population health management, identifying patterns or associations between different factors and health outcomes.

Data normalization

Preprocessing includes normalizing the data to eliminate biases caused by varying scales or distributions. Normalization ensures that features with different ranges contribute equally to the model's learning process. Common normalization techniques include min-max scaling and z-score normalization. For instance, if a dataset contains variables with different scales, such as patient age ranging from 0 to 100 and blood pressure ranging from 80 to 180, normalization techniques such as min-max scaling or log scaling, can be used to bring these variables to a common scale, avoiding bias in model training or evaluation.

Data reduction

Data reduction techniques in AI systems refer to the process of reducing the amount of data or attributes in a dataset while preserving as much of the original dataset's variation as possible. These techniques aim to optimize storage capacity, improve computational efficiency, and enhance the performance of AI models. This can lead to faster training and inference times and improved model interpretability. Here is an example: EHRs contain extensive information about each patient's visit, including clinical notes, lab results, medical history, and more. While comprehensive, this data can be cumbersome for healthcare professionals to review and synthesize.

Using NLP algorithms, key information can be automatically extracted from clinical notes and narratives in the EHR. This could include details like the chief complaint, diagnoses, medications prescribed, procedures performed, etc. The extracted information can be compiled into a condensed summary for each patient visit, which reduces hundreds of pages of EHR data into a succinct overview. As a result, clinicians can more easily review the pertinent details of a patient's case without getting overwhelmed by extraneous data points. This saves healthcare professionals time while allowing them to focus on the most clinically relevant information. The underlying complete EHR still exists if more details are needed. However, for a quick summary, the extracted key data gives clinicians the overview they need in a fraction of the time. This reduction in data volume and dimensionality makes patient data much easier to digest while reducing the risk of clinicians missing critical information buried in verbose notes.

Handling imbalanced data

In certain applications, datasets may be imbalanced, meaning that one class or category is significantly more prevalent than others. Preprocessing techniques, such as oversampling or undersampling, can address this issue by balancing the representation of different classes, preventing biases in model training and evaluation. To illustrate, if a dataset contains patient records with a rare disease, oversampling techniques can generate synthetic data points to balance the representation of that disease class, ensuring that the model does not favor the majority class and can accurately learn from the available data.

Handling missing data

In many data sets, some of the data may be missing. For example, during a patient visit, the patient was not weighed, or his blood pressure was not measured. There are several methods for handling this missing data. These include:

- Deletion: If the amount of missing data is relatively small, the rows or columns containing missing values may be removed. This approach is suitable when missing values are randomly distributed and their removal does not significantly affect the analysis or model performance.
- Mean/mode/median imputation: In this method, missing values are replaced with the mean, mode, or median value of the corresponding feature. This approach assumes that the missing values are missing at random and that the imputed values are representative of the data.
- Forward/backward fill: Also known as "last observation carried forward" or "next observation carried backward," this method involves filling missing values with the previous or subsequent non-missing values in the dataset. It is commonly used in time series data where missing values are expected to have similar patterns to the adjacent values.
- Interpolation: Interpolation methods estimate missing values based on the values of neighboring data points. Common interpolation techniques include linear interpolation, polynomial interpolation, and spline interpolation.
- Multiple imputation: Multiple imputations generate multiple plausible values for each missing data point based on the observed data's distribution. The missing values are then replaced with these imputed values and the analysis is performed multiple times using each imputed dataset. This method accounts for uncertainty in imputation and produces more robust results.

- Model-based imputation: Model-based imputation involves creating a predictive model using the observed data and then using the model to predict missing values. This approach considers the relationships between variables and can provide more accurate imputations.

Handling outliers

Data outliers can have a significant impact on statistical analyses, as they can skew the results and affect the interpretation of the data. For example, a data outlier may be a patient's blood pressure reading of 260/155 when the patient's usual readings are normotensive. Outliers can influence measures such as the mean and standard deviation, leading to biased estimates and misleading conclusions about the data. Therefore, outliers need to be addressed before they are entered into an AI database. Methods for addressing outliers are similar to methods for handling missing data, which include deletion, transformation, imputation, and binning.

- Deletion: In this method, outliers are simply removed from the dataset. This can be done by either deleting the entire data point or replacing the outlier value with a missing value. However, this approach should be used with caution as it can result in the loss of valuable information if the outliers are meaningful or influential.
- Transformation: Data transformation techniques, such as logarithmic or square root transformation, can be applied to reduce the impact of outliers. By compressing the scale of the data, extreme values are brought closer to the rest of the observations, making them less influential in subsequent analyses.
- Imputation: Outlier values can be replaced with estimated values using imputation techniques such as mean, median, or regression imputation. This approach assumes that the outlier values are measurement errors and replaces them with plausible values based on the remaining data.
- Binning: Binning involves grouping the data into intervals or bins and replacing outlier values with bin boundaries. This approach can be

particularly useful when dealing with continuous variables. However, it may lead to a loss of precision in the data.

Feature extraction

Feature extraction is a process used in data science to transform raw data into a set of derived values or characteristics called "features." These features are relevant inputs that can be utilized to create predictive models or perform pattern recognition tasks. The purpose of feature extraction is to reduce the complexity of the dataset by selecting or creating a subset of features that are most informative for the analysis while removing irrelevant or redundant features. This can improve the performance of machine learning models and reduce computational complexity.

In the context of healthcare, feature extraction involves transforming clinical data into a set of relevant features that can be used for analysis and decision-making. These features can include demographic information, lab test results, vital signs, or specific measurements and attributes derived from the data that are deemed important for the analysis.

An example of feature extraction would be the QRS complex duration in an EKG. The QRS complex represents the electrical activation of the ventricles during a heartbeat. The QRS complex duration provides information about the conduction system of the heart and can be indicative of certain cardiac conditions, such as arrhythmias or bundle branch blocks. By analyzing the QRS complex duration, healthcare professionals and researchers can gain insights, make predictions, and support clinical decision-making.

Feature extraction techniques can vary depending on the specific domain and data type. In healthcare, machine learning and pattern recognition algorithms can be employed to identify and extract relevant features from the raw data. These techniques may involve identifying patterns, relationships, or characteristics within the data that are informative for the analysis. By selecting or creating these features, the data can be represented in a more meaningful and concise manner, facilitating subsequent analysis and modeling.

Ethical considerations

It is necessary to pay attention to ethical considerations when collecting and using healthcare data. Patient data must be anonymized to protect privacy and the use of data must comply with regulations such as the Health Insurance Portability and Accountability Act (HIPAA) in the U.S.

Challenges

Each of these steps comes with its own set of challenges. For instance, data collection can be hindered by privacy concerns and data silos, while preprocessing can be complex due to the high dimensionality and heterogeneity of healthcare data. Feature extraction can also be challenging due to the need for domain expertise and the difficulty in selecting the most relevant features.

Consider a scenario where AI is used to predict the risk of heart disease. Data collection may involve gathering patient demographics (age, gender), lifestyle factors (smoking status, exercise habits), medical history (hypertension, diabetes), and diagnostic tests (cholesterol levels, ECG results). During preprocessing, missing values in the data are handled, outliers are identified and addressed, and formats are standardized. Feature extraction could involve calculating risk scores based on established algorithms using the patient's characteristics and test results. By performing these steps, doctors can use AI to analyze complex healthcare data and generate insights that can assist in clinical decision-making. This process ensures that the data is reliable, consistent, and transformed into meaningful features that contribute to accurate predictions, personalized treatment recommendations, and improved patient outcomes.

Conclusion

High-quality, representative data is crucial for training accurate and unbiased AI algorithms. The thoughtful collection, preprocessing, and extraction of features from healthcare data is a critical undertaking that enables AI systems to generate meaningful and equitable insights. The process begins with identifying and collecting diverse data from sources like electronic health records, wearables, and medical imaging. Next, preprocessing techniques are used to clean, standardize, and normalize the data, handling issues like missing values and outliers. The data is then transformed through methods like one-hot encoding to handle categorical variables. Feature extraction is then performed to derive informative variables that can be input into AI models.

By transforming raw data into reliable, standardized, and informative inputs, data scientists and healthcare professionals can train AI models capable of enhancing clinical decision-making and improving patient outcomes. However, each step comes with unique challenges that must be addressed through rigorous techniques and ethical considerations around privacy and bias. If done properly, the promise of AI in healthcare can be realized, augmenting human intelligence to provide more accurate diagnostics, personalized treatments, and optimized delivery of care. However, this is only achievable with high-quality, representative data that captures the diversity of individuals needing healthcare. While there are challenges, these data preparation steps ultimately enable AI systems to generate valuable insights to enhance clinical decision-making and improve patient outcomes.

Chapter 4

The Benefits and Opportunities of AI in Medicine

Introduction

The field of clinical medicine is undergoing a transformative revolution with the integration of Artificial Intelligence (AI) technologies. AI offers numerous benefits and opportunities for improving patient care and transforming healthcare systems. In this chapter, we will investigate how AI programs can enhance not only clinical medicine but the bureaucratic and administrative side of healthcare organizations, too.

Precision medicine

Precision medicine, also known as personalized medicine, is an approach to healthcare that tailors medical treatment and prevention strategies to the individual characteristics of each patient. It considers factors such as a person's genetic makeup, lifestyle, environment, and specific health conditions to provide more accurate and effective interventions. The goal of precision medicine is to optimize patient outcomes by delivering the right treatment to the right patient at the right time.[1] AI plays a significant role in advancing precision medicine by leveraging computational power and sophisticated algorithms to analyze large amounts of complex data.[2] Here are some examples of how AI can help in precision medicine:

Disease diagnosis and risk assessment

AI algorithms can analyze medical images, genetic data, and patient records to identify patterns and detect early signs of diseases. For instance, AI has been used to improve the accuracy of cancer detection in medical imaging. A notable study published in 2023 in the journal *Prostate Cancer and Prostate Disease* demonstrated the effectiveness of AI in cancer detection,[3] whereby researchers trained a deep learning algorithm to analyze MRI scans of prostate cancer patients. The algorithm was able to accurately identify cancerous regions in the scans, achieving results that were nearly identical to those of experienced radiologists. This study highlighted the potential of AI in assisting radiologists and improving the accuracy of cancer diagnosis.

In another example published in Lancet Digital Health in 2022, researchers developed an AI system that can diagnose skin cancer more accurately than dermatologists.[4] The system, developed by a team from Germany, France, and the U.S., achieved a detection accuracy of 95% for cancerous moles and benign spots in images, while a team of 58 dermatologists achieved an accuracy of 87%. This demonstrates the potential of AI to provide more accurate and reliable diagnoses in dermatology.

Treatment selection and optimization

AI can assist in selecting the most appropriate treatment options for individual patients. By analyzing data from diverse sources, including genomic data, electronic health records, and clinical trial data, AI algorithms can provide insights into which treatments are likely to be effective for specific patients, considering their unique characteristics. In a 2019 volume of eBioMedicine, Garcia-Vidal and others created an AI algorithm to help choose the empiric antibiotics for febrile neutropenic patients.[5] Physicians chose the correct empiric antibiotics only 13% of the time in that institution. The AI program was able to search the electronic medical record of every patient in the hospital every four minutes to find febrile neutropenic patients. Once patients were identified, the AI program would evaluate the patient's medical record for current diagnoses, lab results, prior antibiotic use, host microbiota status, etc. Then, the probability of the patient having a multidrug-resistant infection was predicted, thereby aiding in the determination of the optimal antibiotic choice. The algorithm achieved more than a 95% accuracy rate for its predictions.

Drug discovery and development

AI can accelerate the process of drug discovery by analyzing biological and chemical data. Machine learning algorithms can identify patterns and relationships in molecular structures, predict drug-target interactions, and even propose new drug candidates. This enables the development of more targeted and effective therapies. An example of this is when Takeda Pharmaceutical Co. used AI to identify an experimental psoriasis drug candidate in just six months, selecting it out of thousands of potential molecules using AI and machine learning algorithms.[6]

Patient monitoring and outcome prediction

AI can continuously monitor patients' health data, such as vital signs, genomic data, and lifestyle factors, to predict disease progression, treatment response, and potential adverse events.[7] This information can help healthcare providers intervene proactively and personalize treatment plans for better patient outcomes. One example of using AI to continuously monitor patients' health data for predicting disease progression and treatment response is the application of data-driven cluster analysis in diabetes management. Swedish researchers have identified five subgroups of diabetes patients with differences in the risk of disease progression and complications using data-driven cluster analysis.[8] By continuously monitoring patients' health data, including glucose levels, vital signs, lifestyle factors, and genomic data, AI algorithms can analyze patterns and identify the subgroup to which a patient belongs. This information can then be used by the healthcare team to personalize treatment plans, predict disease progression, and assess treatment response.

Precision oncology

AI is being extensively used in oncology to guide treatment decisions based on an individual's tumor characteristics. AI algorithms can analyze genomic data from cancer patients to identify specific genetic alterations and match them with targeted therapies or clinical trials, leading to more precise and personalized cancer treatments.

An example of a place where AI is used to guide treatment decisions in oncology based on tumor characteristics is the Memorial Sloan Kettering Cancer Center (MSKCC) in New York City, United States. MSKCC has developed an AI-driven platform called MSK-IMPACT (Integrated Mutation Profiling of Actionable Cancer Targets).[9] This platform analyzes the genomic data of cancer patients, including DNA sequencing of tumor samples, to identify specific genetic alterations and mutations in their tumors. Using AI algorithms and machine learning techniques, MSK-IMPACT matches these genetic alterations with targeted therapies or relevant clinical trials available at the center. By integrating AI into the analysis and interpretation of genomic data, MSKCC aims to provide oncologists with more precise and personalized treatment options for their patients. The AI algorithms help identify potential treatment options that may be effective based on the unique genetic profile of each patient's tumor. This approach allows for targeted therapy selection, improving the chances of treatment response and overall patient outcomes.

Remote patient care

AI-powered devices and applications can enable remote monitoring of patients, providing real-time feedback and personalized recommendations for managing chronic conditions.[10] This can improve patient engagement, adherence to treatment plans, and overall health outcomes.

There are several examples of AI-powered devices and applications that enable remote monitoring of patients and provide real-time feedback and personalized recommendations for managing chronic conditions. Here are a few:

- Biofourmis: Biofourmis is a digital therapeutics company that utilizes AI to monitor patients with chronic conditions such as heart failure, chronic obstructive pulmonary disease (COPD), and diabetes. Their platform combines wearable sensors, AI algorithms, and predictive analytics to collect and analyze patient data, providing personalized insights and interventions to patients and their healthcare providers.
- Current Health: Current Health provides an AI-powered remote patient monitoring platform that is used for a range of conditions, including post-acute care, chronic disease management, and periop-erative care. Their platform integrates wearable sensors, AI analytics, and patient-reported data to continuously monitor patients' vital signs and health status, alerting healthcare providers to any concerning changes and enabling timely interventions.
- Medtronic CareLink: Medtronic's CareLink system allows remote monitoring of patients with cardiac implantable devices such as pace-makers and defibrillators. The system collects data from these devices and uses AI algorithms to analyze the information, providing health-care professionals with actionable insights and alerts regarding the patient's cardiac health.
- Philips HealthSuite: Philips offers a range of remote patient monitor-ing solutions powered by AI and analytics. Their HealthSuite plat-form enables continuous monitoring of patients with various chronic conditions, including heart failure, COPD, and sleep disorders. The system collects data from connected devices and applies AI algo-rithms to detect trends, predict deterioration, and provide personalized recommendations for managing the conditions.

These examples demonstrate how AI-enabled remote monitoring sys-tems are being used to empower patients, improve engagement, and enhance the management of chronic conditions by providing real-time feedback, personalized recommendations, and timely interventions.

Improved diagnosis and early detection

Early detection of diseases leads to timely interventions and better patient outcomes. AI can help identify subtle patterns or biomarkers that may indicate the presence of a disease before symptoms appear. AI algorithms can analyze medical images with greater accuracy and efficiency, aiding in the identification of diseases. To illustrate, in 2016, researchers at Beth Israel Deaconess Medical Center in Boston, Massachusetts, achieved a groundbreaking milestone in the field of medical diagnostics by developing an AI-powered diagnostic program.[12] This program demonstrated impressive accuracy, correctly identifying cancer in pathology slides 92% of the time, just shy of the 96% accuracy achieved by trained pathologists. However, the true power of AI was unveiled when the two methods, AI and human expertise, were combined, resulting in an astounding 99.5% accuracy.

Building on this success, more recent advancements have showcased the potential of AI in medical diagnostics. In December 2018, researchers at Massachusetts General Hospital (MGH) and Harvard's School of Engineering and Applied Sciences reported the development of a system that rivaled the accuracy of trained radiologists in diagnosing intracranial hemorrhages.[13] Furthermore, in May 2019, researchers at Google and several academic medical centers introduced an AI designed to detect lung cancer with an impressive accuracy of 94%.[14] This AI system outperformed six radiologists, exhibiting both fewer false positives and false negatives.

These achievements highlight the transformative impact of AI in medical diagnostics. The integration of AI algorithms with medical expertise enables enhanced accuracy and efficiency in diagnosing diseases. AI's ability to analyze complex medical images, such as X-rays, MRIs, and CT scans, rivals or surpasses human experts. By processing large amounts of patient data and identifying patterns, AI systems provide valuable support to healthcare professionals, leading to earlier and more accurate diagnoses.

Enhanced healthcare efficiency and cost-effectiveness

Healthcare providers and staff are increasingly burdened by administrative tasks,[15–17] but understanding task patterns and optimizing resource allocation has been challenging due to limited access to meaningful, system-wide data.

The advancement of task management tools in electronic health record systems and the broader adoption of software-as-a-service-based task management systems have opened opportunities to generate more data on tasks and their patterns across users and time. For example, task management systems that manage general tasks, such as Asana or Trello for project management, have helped reduce task complexity and lead to more efficient task completion.[18] This wider availability of data paves the way for leveraging advanced AI algorithms to learn and improve workflows and systems, ultimately aiming to reduce administrative task burden for healthcare providers and organizations, allowing them to focus more on patient care.

In today's healthcare landscape, the digital transformation wave is sweeping across various aspects of hospital operations, not just clinical decision-making. The use of digital technologies has shown promise in helping hospitals make better decisions in areas such as patient flow management, staffing, scheduling, and supply chain management. By harnessing digital transformation, hospitals can enhance the quality and efficiency of care while improving patients' access to it.[19] Moreover, big data analytics plays a crucial role in healthcare organizations.[19,20] The knowledge gained from these programs allows healthcare managers to make informed decisions regarding resource planning, workload measurement, and cost optimization.[21]

The integration of machine learning and stochastic optimization methods can enhance hospital resource planning and scheduling. Stochastic optimization is a technique that incorporates randomness into the optimization process. This allows for the modeling of uncertain real-world variables like variations in patient demand or changes in staff availability.

Machine learning can analyze historical hospital data to forecast future patient volumes and disease patterns. However, forecasts inevitably involve some uncertainty and unpredictability. Stochastic optimization methods explicitly account for this uncertainty in their mathematical models.

Combining machine learning and stochastic optimization enables hospital resource planning under uncertainty. The machine learning forecasts patient workloads and disease trends based on past data. The stochastic optimization then uses these forecasts to generate nurse staffing schedules, operating room timetables, and bed capacity plans while optimizing for efficiency under variability.

This integrated approach provides data-driven scheduling recommendations that are robust to fluctuations in patient demand. The machine learning leverages hospital data patterns while the stochastic optimization handles day-to-day variability. This combination of predictive analytics and uncertainty-aware optimization maximizes resource planning agility in the complex, noisy hospital environment. Streamlined healthcare processes and reduced errors result in cost savings for healthcare systems, which can then be allocated to improving patient care.

The optimization of medical staff workloads and caseload management has become essential for healthcare organizations. By leveraging data analytics, hospitals can improve staffing, and well-being, and enhance patient care.[22] Burnout symptoms due to excessive administrative tasks and long working hours can be mitigated through data-driven approaches that help with staffing optimization, ultimately filling staffing gaps and reducing nurse vacancy rates. The future of healthcare workforce optimization lies in the power of data science. By utilizing advanced analytics techniques, hospitals can better understand and forecast staffing requirements, leading to improved care delivery and cost reduction. Through insightful scheduling, effective labor balance, and increased employee satisfaction, healthcare organizations can create an environment that supports the joy and engagement of the healthcare workforce, ultimately benefiting patients and communities.

In the following paragraphs, we will examine specific examples of how AI can enhance healthcare efficiency and cost-effectiveness.

Health care task management

AI-powered systems can automate administrative tasks in healthcare settings, such as appointment scheduling, documentation, and workflow management.[23] This streamlines operations, reduces paperwork, and frees up healthcare professionals' time for more patient-centered activities. AI-powered systems have been successfully deployed in healthcare settings to automate administrative tasks, resulting in streamlined operations, reduced paperwork, and increased efficiency.

Precision in patient positioning and CT image reconstruction

Radiology departments have utilized AI algorithms to improve precision in patient positioning during CT scans and enhance image reconstruction. This helps ensure consistency in image quality, increases operational efficiency, and improves the overall patient experience.

Administrative workflow assistance

AI has been employed to automate administrative workflows in healthcare organizations. This includes tasks such as appointment scheduling, documentation management, and workflow optimization. By automating these processes, healthcare professionals can save time and focus more on patient-centered activities, leading to improved patient care and satisfaction.

Intelligent automation in revenue cycle management

AI and machine learning have been leveraged to automate various functions in revenue cycle management, such as patient engagement, claims adjudication, risk adjustments, and billing management. By automating these processes, healthcare providers can improve operational efficiency and enhance financial outcomes.

Robotic Process Automation (RPA)

Robotic Process Automation (RPA) refers to the use of software robots or bots to automate repetitive, rule-based tasks in various industries, including healthcare. RPA technology enables the automation of manual processes by mimicking human interactions with digital systems and applications. It can perform tasks such as data entry, data transfer, report generation, and information processing, thereby improving operational efficiency, reducing errors, and freeing up healthcare professionals' time for more complex and value-added activities.[23]

In clinical medicine, RPA has found application in streamlining administrative and operational processes, allowing healthcare organizations to optimize resource allocation, improve patient care, and enhance overall efficiency. One example of RPA use in clinical medicine is the automation of medical billing and claims processing.[24] RPA software can handle tasks such as verifying insurance coverage, processing claims, and generating invoices, reducing the administrative burden on healthcare staff, and improving the accuracy and timeliness of billing processes. Using RPA reduces manual effort, minimizes errors, and accelerates administrative processes.

Chatbots for patient engagement

AI chatbots, also referred to as conversational agents, are software programs designed to simulate typed or verbal conversations with human users, using natural language processing to interpret requests and respond in a human-like manner. AI chatbots are being used to automate patient engagement and education.[25] Chatbots can provide personalized information, answer common questions, and assist with appointment scheduling, freeing up staff time and improving patient experience.

One example of a chatbot being used in clinical medicine is the implementation of chatbots for symptom diagnosis and triage.[26] These chatbots utilize natural language processing (NLP) and AI algorithms to interact with patients, understand their symptoms, and provide appropriate medical advice or direct them to the most suitable healthcare resources. Another notable example is the development of chatbots like Florence,[27] which acts as a personal health assistant and reminder system for patients. Florence, named after Florence Nightingale, the founder of modern nursing, helps patients track their medication schedules, appointments, and activity levels. Another example is the ELIZA chatbot, which was one of the first healthcare chatbots. Developed in 1966 by Joseph Weizenbaum, an MIT computer scientist, ELIZA imitated a psychotherapist and engaged in conversation with users, providing a rudimentary form of mental health support. These chatbots are designed to provide immediate support, offer basic medical advice, and assist in patient triage by asking relevant questions about symptoms and providing appropriate recommendations. They can help alleviate the burden on healthcare providers, improve access to information for patients, and enhance the efficiency of the healthcare system.

Workflow optimization and resource allocation

AI-powered systems can analyze healthcare data to optimize workflow processes and resource allocation.[29] By analyzing patterns and trends, these systems can identify bottlenecks, streamline operations, and ensure efficient utilization of resources, leading to improved productivity and cost savings.

Electronic Health Record (EHR) documentation

AI algorithms can automate the extraction of relevant information from medical documents and populate EHRs.[30,31] This reduces the time and effort required for manual data entry, enhances data accuracy, and improves documentation efficiency.

Medical coding and billing

AI systems can automate medical coding and billing processes by extracting relevant information from clinical notes and assigning appropriate codes.[32] This automation improves coding accuracy, reduces billing errors, and speeds up the reimbursement process.

Expense report auditing

AI can automate the auditing process for employees' expense reports. By analyzing expense data, AI algorithms can identify anomalies, ensure compliance with company policies, and reduce the manual effort required for expense review.

Government operations

AI has the potential to automate administrative tasks in government agencies, such as document processing, data analysis, and citizen services. By automating these processes, governments can improve efficiency, reduce errors, and enhance service delivery to citizens.

HR and compliance

AI can assist in automating administrative tasks in human resources, such as candidate screening, onboarding processes, and compliance monitoring. This improves the employee experience, ensures regulatory compliance, and reduces administrative workloads.

Workflow optimization

AI can analyze and optimize workflows by automating repetitive and rule-based tasks.[33] This includes activities like data entry, form filling, and data processing, leading to increased efficiency and reduced manual effort.

Data analysis and reporting

AI algorithms can automate data analysis and generate reports by extracting insights from large datasets.[34] This eliminates the need for manual data processing, enabling faster and more accurate decision-making.

Email management

AI-powered email management systems can automatically categorize and prioritize incoming emails, filter spam, and suggest appropriate responses.[35] This saves time for employees and improves email productivity.

Data entry and extraction

AI technologies, such as optical character recognition (OCR) and NLP, can automate data entry and extraction from various sources, including documents, forms, and invoices.[36–38] This reduces manual data entry efforts and improves data accuracy.

Virtual assistants and chatbots

AI-powered virtual assistants and chatbots can automate routine administrative tasks, such as answering frequently asked questions, scheduling appointments, and providing basic customer support.[39] This improves customer service and reduces the workload on human staff.

Document management

AI can automate document management processes, including document classification, indexing, and retrieval.[40,41] This enables efficient document organization, easy access to information, and reduces manual effort in handling and managing documents.

Real-time monitoring and predictive analytics

AI-powered systems can monitor patient vital signs continuously and predict deterioration.[42] Imagine wearable devices that can alert healthcare providers to potential emergencies, allowing for proactive interventions and improved outcomes. Early identification of high-risk patients can save lives and reduce hospital readmissions, leading to more efficient healthcare delivery.[43]

Opportunities for AI in clinical medicine

Drug discovery and development

AI can accelerate the drug discovery process by analyzing large amounts of data and identifying potential drug candidates more efficiently. With AI, researchers can uncover new targets for treatments and optimize the efficacy of existing drugs.

Telemedicine and remote patient monitoring

AI-powered virtual consultations and remote monitoring devices enable increased access to healthcare, particularly for patients in remote areas or with limited mobility.[44,45] By overcoming geographical barriers, AI in telemedicine improves patient outcomes and increases convenience for both patients and healthcare providers.

Medical research and data analysis

AI algorithms can analyze large-scale patient data, such as electronic health records and clinical trial data, to extract valuable insights and patterns that may not be readily apparent to humans.[46] This accelerates medical research and facilitates evidence-based decision-making, ultimately leading to improved patient care.

Challenges and limitations of AI in clinical medicine

AI in clinical medicine faces several challenges and limitations that need to be addressed for its successful integration and widespread adoption. These challenges include data quality and interoperability, regulatory and legal considerations, and human-AI collaboration and trust.

Data quality and interoperability

AI relies on high-quality and diverse datasets for training accurate models. Ensuring data availability and compatibility across healthcare systems is a challenge that needs to be addressed. Integrating different data sources and systems can enhance the interoperability of healthcare information, enabling more comprehensive AI applications.

Regulatory and legal considerations

Ethical guidelines and regulations must be established to govern the adoption of AI in clinical settings. These guidelines should address issues such as patient consent, liability, and accountability. Clear frameworks are necessary to ensure the responsible and safe use of AI technologies in healthcare.

Human-AI collaboration and trust

The successful integration of AI in clinical medicine requires a balance between the roles of healthcare professionals and AI algorithms. AI should be seen as a tool to augment human capabilities, not replace them. Building trust and acceptance among clinicians and patients is crucial for the widespread adoption and effective utilization of AI in healthcare.

Conclusion

The integration of AI in clinical medicine offers remarkable benefits and opportunities for improving patient care, personalizing treatments, and enhancing healthcare efficiency. By leveraging AI technologies, healthcare systems can achieve better diagnostic accuracy, early disease detection, and optimized treatment plans. However, it is crucial to address the challenges and ensure the responsible implementation of AI to maximize its potential in clinical medicine. Continued research, development, and collaboration between healthcare professionals and AI systems are necessary for harnessing the full benefits of AI in transforming healthcare.

References

1. Collins FS, Varmus H. (2015) A new initiative on precision medicine. *The New England Journal of Medicine*, **372**(9), 793–795.
2. Ghassemi M, Naumann T, Schulam P, Beam AL, Chen IY, Ranganath R. (2020) A review of challenges and opportunities in machine learning for health. *AMIA Summits on Translational Science Proceedings*, **2020**, 191–200.
3. Chervenkov L, Sirakov N, Kostov G, Velikova T, Hadjidekov G. (2023) Future of prostate imaging: artificial intelligence in assessing prostatic magnetic resonance imaging. *World Journal of Radiology*, **15**(5), 136–145.
4. Columbalia, M, Codella N, *et al.* (2022) Validation of artificial intelligence prediction models for skin cancer diagnosis using dermoscopy images: the 2019

International Skin Imaging Collaboration Grand Challenge. *The Lancet Digital Health*, **4**(5), E330–E339.

5. Garcia-Vidal C, Sanjuan G, Puerta-Alcalde P, Moreno-García E, Soriano A. (2019) Artificial intelligence to support clinical decision-making processes. *EBioMedicine*, **46**, 27–29.

6. Matsuyama K. (2023) AI drug discovery is a $50 billion opportunity for Big Pharma. https://www.bloomberg.com/news/articles/2023-05-09/pharmaceutical-companies-embrace-ai-to-develop-new-drugs?in_source=embedded-checkout-banner

7. Bohr A, Memarzadeh K. (2020) The rise of artificial intelligence in healthcare applications. *Artificial Intelligence in Healthcare*, **2020**, 25–60.

8. Ahlqvist E, Storm P, Käräjämäki A, Martinell M, Dorkhan M, Carlsson A, Vikman P, Prasad RB, Aly DM, Almgren P, Wessman Y, Shaat N, Spégel P, Mulder H, Lindholm E, Melander O, Hansson O, Malmqvist U, Lernmark Å, Lahti K, Forsén T, Tuomi T, Rosengren AH, Groop L. (2018) Novel subgroups of adult-onset diabetes and their association with outcomes: a data-driven cluster analysis of six variables. *The Lancet Diabetes & Endocrinology*, **6**(5), 361–369.

9. Cheng DT, Mitchell TN, Zehir A, Shah RH, Benayed R, Syed A, Chandramohan R, Liu ZY, Won HH, Scott SN, Brannon AR, O'Reilly C, Sadowska J, Casanova J, Yannes A, Hechtman JF, Yao J, Song W, Ross DS, Oultache A, Dogan S, Borsu L, Hameed M, Nafa K, Arcila ME, Ladanyi M, Berger MF. (2015) Memorial Sloan Kettering-integrated mutation profiling of actionable cancer targets (MSK-IMPACT): a hybridization capture-based next-generation sequencing clinical assay for solid tumor molecular oncology. The Journal of Molecular Diagnostics, **17**(3), 251–264.

10. Majumder S, Mondal T, Deen MJ. (2017) Wearable sensors for remote health monitoring. *Sensors (Basel)*, **17**(1), 130.

11. Liu Y, Gadepalli K, Norouzi M, Dahl GE, Kohlberger T, Boyko A, Venugopalan S, Timofeev A, Nelson PQ, Corrado GS, Hipp JD, Peng LH, Stumpe MC. (2017) Detecting cancer metastases on gigapixel pathology images. *ArXiv, abs/1703.02442*

12. Kritz (2016). Artificial intelligence achieves near-human performance in diagnosing breast cancer. https://www.bidmc.org/about-bidmc/news/artificial-intelligence-achieves-near-human-performance-in-diagnosing-breast-cancer

13. Lee H, Yune S, Mansouri M, Kim M, Tajmir SH, Guerrier CE, Ebert SA, Pomerantz SR, Romero JM, Kamalian S, Gonzalez RG, Lev MH, Do S.

(2019) An explainable deep-learning algorithm for the detection of acute intracranial haemorrhage from small datasets. *Nature Biomedical Engineering*, **3**(3), 173–182.

14. Ardila D, Kiraly AP, Bharadwaj S, *et al.* (2019) End-to-end lung cancer screening with three-dimensional deep learning on low-dose chest computed tomography. *Nature Medicine*, **25**, 954–961.

15. Department of Health and Human Services; Health Resources and Services Administration; National Center for Health Workforce Analysis. (2019) Brief summary results from the 2018 National Sample Survey of Registered Nurses. https://data.hrsa.gov/DataDownload/NSSRN/GeneralPUF18/nssrn-summary-report.pdf.

16. Willard-Grace R, Knox M, Huang B, Hammer H, Kivlahan C, Grumbach K. (2019) Burnout and health care workforce turnover. *Annals of Family Medicine*, **17**(1), 36–41.

17. Sinsky C, Colligan L, Li L, Prgomet M, Reynolds S, Goeders L, Westbrook J, Tutty M, Blike G. (2016) Allocation of physician time in ambulatory practice: a time and motion study in 4 specialties. *Annals of Internal Medicine*, **165**(11), 753–760.

18. O'Malley AS, Draper K, Gourevitch R, Cross DA, Scholle SH. (2015) Electronic health records and support for primary care teamwork. *Journal of the American Medical Informatics Association*, **22**, 426–434.

19. Raghupathi W, Raghupathi V. (2014) Big data analytics in healthcare: promise and potential. *Health Information Science and Systems*, **2**, 3.

20. Dash S, Shakyawar SK, Sharma M, *et al.* (2019) Big data in healthcare: management, analysis and future prospects. *Journal of Big Data*, **6**, 54.

21. Batko K, Ślęzak A. (2022) The use of big data analytics in healthcare. *Journal of Big Data*, **9**(1), 3.

22. Kim S, Song H. (2022) How digital transformation can improve hospitals' operational decisions. https://hbr.org/2022/01/how-digital-transformation-can-improve-hospitals-operational-decisions

23. Utermohlen K. (2018) Four robotic process automation (RPA) applications in the healthcare industry. https://medium.com/@karl.utermohlen/4-robotic-process-automation-rpa-applications-in-the-healthcare-industry-4d449b24b613

24. Rosen H. (2023) Using robotic process automation in healthcare: opportunities and obstacles. https://www.forbes.com/sites/forbesbusinesscouncil/2023/06/22/using-robotic-process-automation-in-healthcare-opportunities-and-obstacles/?sh=3ed9e5e46194

25. Laranjo L, *et al.* (2018) Conversational agents in healthcare: a systematic review. *Journal of the American Medical Informatics Association*, **25**(9), 1248–1258.
26. You Y, Gui X. (2021) Self-diagnosis through AI-enabled Chatbot-based Symptom Checkers: user experiences and design considerations. *AMIA Annual Symposium Proceedings*, **2020**, 1354-1363.
27. https://www.florence.chat/#:~:text=Florence%20reminds%20users%20to%20take,to%20present%20medicine%20specific%20information
28. Rossen J. (2023) 'Please Tell Me Your Problem': Remembering ELIZA, the Pioneering '60s Chatbot. https://www.mentalfloss.com/posts/eliza-chatbot-history
29. Letourneau-Guillon L, Camiranda D, Guilbert F, Forghani R. (2020) Artificial intelligence applications for workflow, process optimization, and predictive analytics. *Neuroimaging Clinics of North America*, **30**(4), e1–e15.
30. Natural language processing in healthcare. https://www.foreseemed.com/natural-language-processing-in-healthcare
31. Maiti S. (2023) Extracting medical information from clinical text with NLP. https://www.analyticsvidhya.com/blog/2023/02/extracting-medical-information-from-clinical-text-with-nlp/
32. Dong H, Falis M, Whiteley W, *et al.* (2022) Automated clinical coding: what, why, and where we are? *npj Digital Medicine*, **5**, 159.
33. Understanding artificial intelligence in business. https://www.artsyltech.com/blog/Artificial-Intelligence-in-Business#:~:text=AI%20technologies%20like%20robotic%20process,reduce%20errors%2C%20and%20enhance%20productivity
34. The role of AI and automation for improved data analytics. https://gleematic.com/the-role-of-ai-and-automation-for-improved-data-analytics/
35. Todoros O. (2023) The future of business email: how AI tools will improve your inbox. https://www.spikenow.com/blog/conversational-email/the-future-of-business-email-how-ai-tools-will-improve-your-inbox/
36. Tripathi P. (2023) How AI and deep learning have revolutionized document processing automation. https://www.docsumo.com/blog/document-ai
37. (2023) How AI in healthcare can improve the efficiency of HER systems? https://itechindia.co/us/blog/ai-in-ehr-software-systems-using-ai-to-improve-ehrs-data-in-healthcare/#:~:text=AI%20in%20EHR%20uses%20new,data%20discovery%20and%20personalized%20recommendations.
38. Pandey V. (2022) Unleashing the power of Intelligent Document Processing (IDP) with AI, RPA and OCR. https://www.linkedin.com/pulse/unleashing-power-intelligent-document-processing-idp-ai-pandey-/

39. Krzysztof M. (2020) Chatbots in healthcare: benefits, risks, and 5 insightful use cases. https://codete.com/blog/chatbots-in-healthcare

40. Saitwal A. (2022) Why is it essential to have automated document indexing? https://www.klearstack.com/essential-to-have-automated-document-indexing/

41. Sarma R. (2023) The future of Artificial Intelligence in document management systems. https://www.linkedin.com/pulse/future-artificial-intelligence-document-management-systems-sarma/

42. Kennedy S. (2022) Patient deterioration predictor outperforms vital sign measurements. https://healthitanalytics.com/news/patient-deterioration-predictor-outperforms-vital-sign-measurements

43. Romero-Brufau S, Wyatt KD, Boyum P, Mickelson M, Moore M, Cognetta-Rieke C. (2020) Implementation of Artificial Intelligence-based clinical decision support to reduce hospital readmissions at a regional hospital. *Applied Clinical Informatics*, **11**(4), 570–577.

44. Cho KJ, Kwon O, Kwon JM, Lee Y, Park H, Jeon KH, Kim KH, Park J, Oh BH. (2020) detecting patient deterioration using Artificial Intelligence in a rapid response system. *Critical Care Medicine*, **48**(4), e285–e289.

45. Telemedicine technology powered by AI and IoT. https://www.intel.com/content/www/us/en/healthcare-it/telemedicine.html

46. Askin S, Burkhalter D, Calado G, El Dakrouni S. (2023) Artificial Intelligence applied to clinical trials: opportunities and challenges. Health and Technology, **13**(2), 203–213.

Chapter 5

Machine Learning

Introduction

Machine learning has emerged as a transformative technology in various industries, including clinical medicine. In this chapter, we will explore the concept of machine learning, its relationship with AI, and its relevance to healthcare professionals.

What is machine learning?

Machine learning (ML), a subset of artificial intelligence (AI), allows systems to learn and improve from past experiences without the need for explicit programming. In essence, ML algorithms find patterns or regularities in data.[1] The concept of ML in data science involves using statistical learning and optimization methods to analyze datasets and identify patterns.[2] Now, to better understand this, consider a simple analogy. Imagine teaching a child to differentiate between apples and oranges. Initially, the child might make mistakes, but with repeated exposure and corrections, the child starts identifying them correctly. ML works similarly, but instead of fruits, it learns by using data.

How machine learning works

ML algorithms can learn from data and make predictions without explicit programming. By analyzing large datasets and identifying patterns, ML models can generate insights that support clinical decision-making, improve patient outcomes, and enhance medical research. A key aspect of ML is the ability to train the algorithms using labeled data. Labeled data consists of input samples paired with their corresponding outputs, such as medical images with known diagnoses. During the training process, the algorithm learns to recognize patterns in the data and adjusts its internal parameters to optimize its predictions. For example, an algorithm trained on a dataset of mammograms without cancer and a set with corresponding breast cancer diagnoses can learn to detect suspicious features in new mammograms and predict the likelihood of cancer. These algorithms can discover relationships in data that have eluded scientists in the past.

In a study published in the Journal of Medical Internet Research, entitled *Impact of Big Data Analytics on People's Health: Overview of Systematic Reviews and Recommendations for Future Studies*,[3] researchers developed a model that assimilated multiple types of a patient's health data, including symptoms, biometric data, lab tests, and body scans, to aid doctors in making decisions with incomplete information. The model utilized ML techniques to predict disease risks and design personalized treatment plans. The researchers found that the use of big data analytics has demonstrated moderate to high accuracy in diagnosing certain diseases, managing chronic diseases, and supporting real-time analysis of large datasets for predicting disease outcomes. Similarly, researchers from MIT have developed a ML model that improves the prediction of patient mortality in intensive care units (ICUs) during their first two days of admission.[4] The model analyzes physiological data from electronic health records of previously admitted ICU patients, including those who died during their stay. By examining factors such as heart rate, blood pressure, lab test results (including glucose levels and white blood cell count), and other indicators, the model identifies high predictors of mortality. It then categorizes patients into subpopulations based on their health status. This analysis allows the model to learn patterns and associations between physiological data and the likelihood of death in the following 48 hours. When a new patient arrives, the model can examine their physiological data from the first 24 hours and utilize the knowledge gained from analyzing patient subpopulations to provide a more accurate estimation of the patient's likelihood of dying in the following 48 hours. By leveraging the insights gained from previous cases, the model enhances mortality prediction for new patients in the critical early stages of their ICU stay. This approach improves upon traditional scoring systems by incorporating ML techniques and analyzing patient subpopulations. Unlike "global" models trained on a single large patient population or models that focus on limited subpopulations, the proposed model combines the advantages of both approaches. It trains on specific patient subpopulations but also shares data across all subpopulations to improve predictions. The model's ability to assess the likelihood of death based on the first 24 hours of data addresses the need for timely and accurate predictions, which can assist healthcare providers in making informed decisions regarding patient care in the ICU. The unique aspect of this model is that it combines training on patient subpopulations with data sharing across all subpopulations, resulting in more accurate predictions compared to strictly global or other models. Evaluating the model by specific subpopulations also reveals performance disparities of the more commonly employed global models in predicting mortality across different patient groups, providing valuable insights for developing more accurate models tailored to specific patients. The goal is to identify patients who are at immediate risk and require immediate attention in ICUs.

What is feature extraction?

ML algorithms work by detecting patterns in the data to make predictions or classifications. The raw data that is fed into a ML algorithm can often be very complex and contain lots of details that are irrelevant for the task at hand. For example, an image recognition algorithm does not need to analyze every single pixel in an image, it just needs to identify the key features like edges, shapes, and textures that are useful for determining what object is in the image. This is where feature extraction comes in. Feature extraction is the process of transforming the raw data into a reduced set of variables or "features" that are useful for the learning task and algorithms.[5]

For images, this could mean extracting features like color histograms, line and edge detections, textures, etc. For audio data, it could mean extracting spectral features related to tone and pitch. The goal is to extract information that is meaningful while discarding excess noise and redundancy. The selected features serve as inputs to the ML algorithms, enabling them to learn the relationships between the features and the desired outcomes.

How does feature extraction help machine learning algorithms?

Feature extraction is an important part of preparing medical data for machine learning algorithms. It transforms the raw patient data into a condensed set of variables that expose the most relevant information. For example, a heart disease prediction algorithm may extract features like cholesterol level, blood pressure trends, smoking status, rather than analyzing every single data point from an EKG readout. This reduces the complexity for the algorithm to find meaningful patterns. It also focuses the algorithm on the most useful clinical factors for predicting heart disease risk, rather than getting distracted by irrelevant variances in the data. Through techniques like standardizing test result scales and normalizing distributions, feature extraction can make it easier for the algorithm to detect health risk patterns across patient populations. Additionally, reducing the raw data down to key features decreases the risk of overfitting to inconsequential fluctuations and noise in the data. Overall, thoughtful feature engineering ensures that algorithms learn from meaningful relationships in medical data, not incidental variations. This facilitates more accurate predictions to aid healthcare professionals in tasks like diagnosis and treatment planning.

Testing machine learning models

ML models are constructed using various algorithms that suit the specific task and dataset. These models capture the learned patterns from the training data and can be applied to make predictions on new, unseen data. To evaluate the model's performance, it is tested on a separate dataset, often referred to as a "validation set" or "test set" with known outcomes.

Here is a hypothetical example of how a validation set would be used in medicine. A research team developed a machine learning model to predict hospital readmission risk for patients with heart failure. They collected data on thousands of heart failure patients including their demographics, medications, lab results, procedures, and whether they were readmitted within 30 days of discharge. The researchers split the dataset into a training set (80% of the data) to train the model and a test set (20% of the data) to evaluate it. The training data was used to tune the model parameters and capture patterns that are predictive of readmission. Once the model was trained, they evaluated its performance by running the test set through the model and comparing its readmission predictions to the actual observed outcomes for those patients. Metrics like accuracy, precision, recall, F1 score, and area under receiver operating characteristic curve (AUC) were used to quantify prediction accuracy. This allows them to objectively measure how well the model generalizes to new patients. The model performance on the test set gives a reliable estimate of its real-world performance when deployed clinically. Evaluating on an independent test set prevents overfitting and ensures the model is robust.

Domains of machine learning

ML is one of the key techniques used to achieve AI capabilities. AI encompasses a broader scope, aiming to create intelligent systems that can mimic human intelligence in various tasks. ML algorithms provide the foundation for many AI applications by enabling systems to learn and improve from experience. In a healthcare setting, ML algorithms can improve performance in the following domains:

- **Diagnosis and prognosis**: ML algorithms can analyze patient data, including medical records, imaging scans, and laboratory results, to assist physicians in diagnosing diseases and predicting outcomes. For instance, researchers have developed ML models that accurately predict the risk of certain cancers based on patient characteristics and biomarkers.[6] These models can help physicians identify high-risk patients and tailor treatment plans accordingly.
- **Drug discovery and personalized medicine**: ML plays a crucial role in drug discovery by analyzing vast datasets to identify potential drug candidates and predict their efficacy.[7] By integrating genetic

information, clinical data, and treatment outcomes, ML algorithms can also enable personalized medicine, tailoring treatments to individual patients based on their unique characteristics and responses to therapy.

- **Clinical decision support**: ML models can act as intelligent decision support tools, providing physicians with evidence-based recommendations and predictions.[8,9] For example, algorithms can analyze patient symptoms, medical history, and test results to assist in differential diagnosis and suggest appropriate treatment options. This can help reduce diagnostic errors, improve treatment outcomes, and enhance efficiency in healthcare delivery.

- **Image analysis and radiology**: ML algorithms excel in image analysis tasks, aiding radiologists in the interpretation of medical images such as X-rays, CT scans, and MRIs.[10,11] These algorithms can assist in the detection of abnormalities, segmentation of structures, and quantification of disease progression. By automating certain image analysis tasks, ML can save time for physicians and improve diagnostic accuracy.

How do machine learning algorithms use data to make predictions?

At the heart of ML is the concept of training data. Training data refers to the large sets of labeled or unlabeled data used to train ML models. These data are used to teach the AI algorithms how to recognize patterns, make predictions, or perform specific tasks. In the case of healthcare, these data could include patient records, medical images, lab test results, and other relevant information. The quality and quantity of training data significantly impact the performance and generalization of the AI model. The training process involves feeding this data into the ML algorithm, which then learns from it by identifying patterns and relationships. The algorithm uses various mathematical techniques to extract meaningful features from the data and builds a model that captures the underlying patterns. Once the model is trained, it can be used to make predictions or identify patterns in new, unseen data. For example, for a ML model trained in predicting the likelihood of a patient developing a particular disease, the patient's relevant data can be input into the model to obtain a prediction.

The key idea behind ML is that the algorithm learns from the data rather than being explicitly programmed. This allows the algorithm to discover complex relationships and patterns that may not be apparent to humans. For example, researchers from Google and Stanford University used deep learning algorithms to analyze retinal fundus images and identify patients at risk for major cardiovascular events, like heart attacks and strokes.[12] By looking at the retinal blood vessels, the ML model was able to detect subtle patterns in vessel topology and branching that correlated with cardiovascular risk factors. These were complex patterns that human clinicians would unlikely consistently identify from visual inspection alone. The deep learning algorithm was trained on data from 284,335 patients and validated on two independent datasets. It was able to predict cardiovascular risk factors such as age, gender, smoking status, and major cardiac events. The AUC for predicting major cardiac events was 0.70, comparable to other scoring systems.

It is important to note that while very impressive in some respects, ML algorithms are not infallible and their predictions may not always be accurate. However, with proper training and validation, these algorithms can provide valuable insights and assist in clinical decision-making.

Types of machine learning algorithms

ML algorithms offer valuable capabilities in healthcare, including supervised learning for medical diagnosis, unsupervised learning for patient clustering, and reinforcement learning for treatment optimization, ultimately improving patient outcomes and personalized care.

Supervised learning

Supervised learning algorithms are ML algorithms that learn from labeled data and aim to make predictions on new, unlabeled instances. In healthcare, these algorithms can be used for medical diagnosis by training them on historical patient data with known diagnoses. This allows the algorithms to analyze new patient data, such as symptoms, medical history, and test results, and predict the most likely diagnosis or provide risk assessments.

Unsupervised learning

Unsupervised learning algorithms analyze unlabeled data and seek to identify patterns or group similar instances without predefined labels. In healthcare, these algorithms are valuable for tasks such as clustering patient data. By applying unsupervised learning algorithms like k-means clustering or hierarchical clustering to vast amounts of patient data, healthcare professionals can group patients with similar characteristics or conditions. This clustering helps identify subpopulations, patterns, or phenotypes within the patient data, leading to personalized treatment strategies, targeted interventions, or a better understanding of disease subtypes.

Reinforcement algorithms

Reinforcement learning algorithms learn through interactions with an environment and receive feedback in the form of rewards or penalties. In a healthcare context, reinforcement learning can be used to optimize treatment decisions and improve patient outcomes. For example, by simulating different treatment options, observing the patient's response, and receiving rewards or penalties based on health outcomes, reinforcement learning algorithms can learn the optimal treatment strategy for individual patients.

These different types of ML algorithms offer valuable capabilities in healthcare, enabling tasks such as diagnosis, patient clustering, and treatment optimization. The adoption of ML in healthcare is increasing, with numerous applications being explored and developed to improve patient care and outcomes. For a more complete discussion of the types of ML algorithms, see Chapter 2.

Types of data used by machine learning algorithms

In a healthcare setting, ML algorithms leverage various types of data to improve medical diagnostics, treatment planning, disease prediction, and patient outcomes. The types of data commonly used in healthcare ML applications include electronic health records, medical images, and genomic data.

Electronic Health Records (EHRs)

EHRs contain a wealth of patient information, including demographic data, medical history, laboratory results, medications, and clinical notes. ML models can analyze EHR data to predict disease risks, identify patterns in patient outcomes, and support clinical decision-making. However, challenges arise due to the heterogeneity and complexity of EHR data, including missing values, unstructured text, and inconsistencies in data entry. Data preprocessing and cleaning are essential to ensure data quality and improve the performance of ML models.

Medical images

Medical imaging techniques such as X-rays, CT scans, MRI, and histopathology slides provide valuable visual information for diagnosis and treatment planning. ML algorithms, particularly deep learning models, can analyze medical images to detect abnormalities, classify diseases, and segment anatomical structures. For example, deep learning algorithms have demonstrated success in detecting diabetic retinopathy from retinal fundus photographs and identifying lymph node metastases from breast cancer histopathology slides. However, the large size of medical image datasets and the need for expert annotations pose challenges in terms of data acquisition, annotation, and computational requirements for training deep learning models.

Genomic data

Genomic data, which includes DNA sequences, gene expression profiles, and genetic variations, plays a crucial role in personalized medicine and understanding the genetic basis of diseases. ML algorithms can analyze genomic data to identify genetic markers, predict disease risks, and guide treatment selection. However, genomic data is high-dimensional with many features and often exhibits complex relationships. Preprocessing genomic data, addressing issues such as missing values and batch effects, and selecting informative features are important steps to ensure accurate and reliable predictions.

Challenges in using clinical data in machine learning algorithms

Using clinical data in ML algorithms presents several challenges that need to be addressed to ensure accurate and reliable outcomes.

Quality of data

One of the main challenges is the quality and availability of clinical data. Clinical data is often complex, heterogeneous, and stored in various formats, making it challenging to aggregate and preprocess for analysis. Data quality issues such as missing values, inconsistencies, and biases can impact the performance and generalizability of ML models, leading to biased and unreliable results.

Data integration

Another challenge is the integration of clinical data from different sources. Data integration poses a significant challenge in healthcare due to the diverse sources of clinical data. Healthcare systems generate vast amounts of data, including EHRs, medical imaging, genomic information, and physiologic data from wearable devices. Integrating and harmonizing these data sources is essential for comprehensive analysis and deriving meaningful insights.

The problem with data integration arises from the volume, velocity, and variety of the data. The sheer volume of data makes it difficult to manage and process effectively. Additionally, the data comes from various sources at different speeds, leading to challenges in capturing and processing it in a timely manner. Moreover, the variety of data formats and structures complicates the integration process. To solve the problem of data integration, robust data management strategies and interoperability standards are required. Organizations need to implement data governance frameworks and establish data integration best practices. These practices involve consolidating data from disparate sources into a single source of truth, where data can be transformed and shared. Various technologies and tools are available to facilitate data integration, such as Extract, Transform, Load (ETL) processes, application programming interfaces (APIs), and data integration platforms.

By implementing effective data management strategies, organizations can overcome data integration challenges and leverage the full potential of diverse clinical data sources in healthcare.

Data quality and standardization

Ensuring the quality, completeness, and standardization of data across different healthcare systems and institutions is a challenge. Variations in data formats, coding schemes, and data entry practices can introduce noise and inconsistencies, affecting the performance of ML models.

Privacy and security

Healthcare data, particularly EHRs and genomic data, contain sensitive and personally identifiable information. Protecting patient privacy and ensuring data security are critical concerns. Complying with privacy regulations, such as the Health Insurance Portability and Accountability Act (HIPAA) in the United States, implementing robust data encryption techniques, and employing secure data-sharing protocols are necessary to maintain patient confidentiality.

Interpretability and explainability

Furthermore, the interpretability and explainability of ML models are crucial in the clinical domain. Healthcare professionals need to understand the reasoning behind the model's predictions and decisions to build trust and ensure the models are aligned with clinical guidelines. Black-box models may hinder the acceptance and adoption of ML solutions in clinical practice.

Data imbalance and bias

Healthcare datasets can suffer from class imbalance, where certain rare conditions or outcomes are underrepresented. A class imbalance occurs when there is a significant disparity in the number of instances between different classes or categories within the dataset. Classes can include: diagnosis codes, procedure codes, demographic information, vital signs, etc. This can lead to biased models that perform well in the majority class but poorly on the minority class. Addressing data imbalance and mitigating bias in training data is important to ensure fair and accurate predictions.

Ethical considerations

Ethical considerations and bias mitigation are also critical challenges in using clinical data. ML algorithms are susceptible to inherent biases present in the data, which can lead to disparities in diagnosis, treatment, and outcomes among different patient populations. Ensuring fairness, transparency, and equity in the development and deployment of ML models is essential for ethical and unbiased clinical decision-making.

Updating data

The dynamic nature of healthcare introduces challenges in maintaining the performance and generalizability of ML models over time. The models need to be continuously updated and validated to account for changes in patient populations, clinical guidelines, and evolving healthcare practices.

Despite these challenges, ML in healthcare holds great promise for improving patient care, accelerating medical research, and enhancing healthcare decision-making. Ongoing research and collaboration between data scientists, healthcare providers, and policymakers are essential to overcome these challenges and unlock the full potential of ML in healthcare.

Application areas of machine learning in clinical medicine

ML has found numerous application areas in clinical medicine, including image analysis, predictive modeling, and decision support systems. These applications leverage the power of ML algorithms to extract meaningful insights from medical data and improve patient care. Here are some real-world examples of these algorithms:

Image analysis

ML algorithms are used to analyze medical images and aid in the diagnosis, segmentation, and detection of abnormalities. For instance, in radiology, deep learning models have been developed to detect lung nodules in chest X-rays and CT scans and to identify lesions in brain MRI scans. These algorithms help radiologists improve accuracy and efficiency in image interpretation.

Predictive modeling

ML techniques enable predictive modeling to estimate patient outcomes, disease risks, and treatment responses. For example, predictive models based on ML have been developed to forecast disease progression in conditions like diabetes, cardiovascular diseases, and cancer. These models use patient data such as demographics, medical history, and laboratory results to predict future health outcomes. They assist clinicians in making informed decisions and designing personalized treatment plans.

Decision support systems

ML algorithms can serve as decision support systems by providing recommendations or assisting clinicians in making critical decisions. These systems utilize patient data and clinical guidelines to offer personalized treatment suggestions. An example is the use of ML algorithms in oncology to recommend optimal treatment options based on patient characteristics, tumor characteristics, and treatment response data. Decision support systems enhance clinical decision-making and improve patient outcomes.

These are just a few examples of how ML is applied in clinical medicine. ML algorithms are also used for predicting adverse events, optimizing patient scheduling, analyzing electronic health records, and improving clinical trial design. The applications continue to expand as researchers and healthcare professionals explore the potential of ML in various medical domains.

References

1. Rao SVA, *et al.* (2017) A survey on machine learning: concept, algorithms, and applications. https://www.smec.ac.in/assets/images/committee/research/17-18/282.A%20Survey%20on%20Machine%20Learning%20Concept,.pdf
2. Brown s. (2021) Maching learning, explained. https://mitsloan.mit.edu/ideas-made-to-matter/machine-learning-explained
3. Borges do Nascimento IJ, Marcolino MS, Abdulazeem HM, Weerasekara I, Azzopardi-Muscat N, Gonçalves MA, Novillo-Ortiz D. (2021) Impact of big data analytics on people's health: overview of systematic reviews and recommendations for future studies. *Journal of Medical Internet Research*, **23**(4), e27275.
4. Matheson R. (2018) Model improves prediction of mortality risk in ICU patients. https://news.mit.edu/2018/model-improves-prediction-mortality-risk-icu-patients-0829
5. Feature extraction. https://deepai.org/machine-learning-glossary-and-terms/feature-extraction
6. Al-Tashi Q, Saad MB, Muneer A, Qureshi R, Mirjalili S, Sheshadri A, Le X, Vokes NI, Zhang J, Wu J. (2023) Machine learning models for the identification of prognostic and predictive cancer biomarkers: a systematic review. *International Journal of Molecular Sciences*, **24**(9), 7781.
7. Dara S, Dhamercherla S, Jadav SS, Babu CM, Ahsan MJ. (2022) Machine learning in drug discovery: a review. *Artificial Intelligence Review*, **55**(3), 1947–1999.

8. Giordano C, Brenna M, *et al.* (2021) Accessing artificial intelligence for clinical decision-making. *Frontiers in Digital Health*, **3**, 645232.
9. Basu R, Archer N, Mukherjee B. (2012) Intelligent decision support in healthcare. https://pubsonline.informs.org/do/10.1287/LYTX.2012.01.05/full/
10. Hosny A, Parmar C, Quackenbush J, Schwartz LH, Aerts HJWL. (2018) Artificial intelligence in radiology. *Nature Reviews Cancer*, **18**(8):500–510.
11. Wang S, Summers RM. (2012) Machine learning and radiology. *Medical Image Analysis*, **16**(5), 933–951.
12. Poplin R, Varadarajan AV, Blumer K, *et al.* (2018) Prediction of cardiovascular risk factors from retinal fundus photographs via deep learning. *Nature Biomedical Engineering*, **2**, 158–164.

Chapter 6

Limitations in Algorithmic Generalizability

Introduction

Artificial Intelligence (AI) has the potential to revolutionize the field of medicine, offering new opportunities to improve patient outcomes, enhance the delivery of care, and advance medical research. However, the use of AI in medicine is not without challenges. One significant challenge is the limited generalizability of AI models, which hinders their seamless translation into clinical practice.[1] Generalizability refers to the ability of AI models to perform accurately on new data that differs from its initial training data. In other words, AI models can apply their learned knowledge to different patient populations, diverse healthcare settings, and varied disease presentations and arrive at correct diagnoses and recommendations. The limitations in generalizability pose obstacles to the widespread adoption and effective implementation of AI techniques in real-world clinical scenarios.

To illustrate this challenge, consider a doctor who has just diagnosed a patient with cancer. The doctor is aware of recent advances in AI and its potential to personalize treatment based on genetic subtypes of the disease. However, for the AI model to provide accurate recommendations, it needs to have been trained on a large and diverse dataset that represents various genetic backgrounds, ethnicities, and disease subtypes. If the AI model was primarily trained on a limited population or lacked diversity in its training data, it may not generalize well to the patient's specific case, compromising the accuracy of treatment recommendations.

The limitations in the generalizability of AI models in medicine can arise due to several factors, such as biased or incomplete training data, data quality issues, and the dynamic nature of healthcare practice. Addressing these challenges requires careful consideration in the development and evaluation of AI models, as well as ongoing monitoring and validation in real-world clinical settings.

In this chapter, we will delve deeper into the concept of limited generalizability in AI for medicine and explore its implications for health professionals. We will discuss the factors contributing to limited generalizability and its impact on clinical decision-making. Furthermore, we will explore strategies and best practices to enhance the generalizability of AI models and promote their successful integration into healthcare workflows. By gaining a comprehensive understanding of these challenges, health professionals can effectively harness the power of AI while ensuring patient safety and improving healthcare outcomes.

Causes of lack of generalizability

Causes of a lack of generalizability in medical AI models can vary and may include the following:

Limited diversity in training data

If the AI model is trained on a dataset that is not representative of the diverse population or healthcare settings in which it will be deployed, it may struggle to generalize its findings.[2] Machine learning algorithms rely heavily on their training data. If the training data is not sufficiently diverse and representative, it can lead to biases and poor generalizability when the model is deployed. For example, if the algorithm is only trained on data from a single healthcare system, it may fail to account for differences across other health systems. The patient populations, disease patterns, and clinical practices often vary between health systems, limiting the portability of algorithms trained on data from just one system. Similarly, if the training data only includes patients from a single geographic region, the algorithm may not generalize well to other areas with different patient demographics, disease prevalence, and incidence rates. To improve generalizability, machine learning models need to be trained on diverse, multi-site datasets that capture a wide range of patient populations, disease patterns, and clinical practice variations.

Differences in data collection protocols

Variations in data collection methods, equipment, or imaging techniques across different healthcare settings can impact the generalizability of AI models trained on specific datasets.[3] Institutional differences limit the ability to generalize the performance of an AI algorithm validated at one site to new settings. An AI model that performs well when tested in the institution where it was developed may struggle to maintain the same performance when deployed in new hospitals with different equipment, workflows, and patient demographics. For more robust evaluation and development, AI algorithms need to be trained and validated on diverse multi-site data that captures a wide range of institutional variations. This can improve generalizability and enable a more accurate assessment of expected performance when an algorithm is applied clinically across different healthcare systems.

Contextual variations

Medical AI models designed to interpret diagnostic images, predict diseases, or recommend treatments may encounter different clinical practices, guidelines, and protocols across healthcare institutions or regions. This can limit generalizability if the model is only trained on data from a specific context. For example, an AI model trained on chest X-ray images from one hospital may not perform well on X-rays from other sites with different imaging equipment, techniques, or aquisition protocols. A model trained on disease diagnoses or treatment decisions based on one institution's specific diagnostic criteria, preferred interventions, referral availability, and data capture methods may fail to generalize well to new healthcare systems with different populations, resources, and workflows. For example, an AI model trained to diagnose diseases like pneumonia or

COVID-19 based on one institution's specific diagnostic guidelines may not generalize well to institutions with slightly different diagnostic thresholds or criteria. The key challenge is that clinical practices and standards vary considerably, so for robust performance, AI models need sufficiently diverse and multi-context training data representing a wide range of real-world medical environments, as opposed to data from just a single institution. Capturing multi-site variabilities during training is essential for developing highly generalizable AI.

Bias in the training data

Biases in the data used to train AI models can result in limited generalizability. If the training data is biased towards certain demographic groups or lacks diversity, the model may not perform well when applied to other populations, leading to disparities in outcomes.

Overfitting

Overfitting refers to a situation in machine learning where an algorithm becomes too closely tailored to the training data, resulting in a poor ability to generalize to new data.[4] When a model overfits, it fits the training data extremely well, including any noise or random fluctuations present in the data. However, this excessive focus on the training data can lead to a loss of predictive power when applied to unseen data. In other words, overfitting occurs when a model becomes too complex or intricate, trying to capture every detail and idiosyncrasy of the training data. Imagine a scenario where a machine learning model is being developed to predict the likelihood of patients developing diabetes based on their medical records. The dataset includes a wide range of factors such as age, weight, height, blood pressure, family history, as well as more subtle details like the number of visits to the doctor, types of medications taken in the past, and various laboratory test results. If the model is excessively complex and is trained on a limited amount of patient data, it may start to identify and rely on spurious correlations that happen to appear in the training dataset but do not hold in general. For example, the model might pick up that a small group of patients who visited a particular healthcare provider and were prescribed a specific medication later developed diabetes. The model could erroneously learn that these are important predictive features when, in fact, they are coincidental and not causally related to the onset of diabetes. As a result, the model may not be able to capture the underlying patterns and relationships that would enable it to make accurate predictions on new, unseen data. To safeguard against overfitting in medical machine learning applications, healthcare professionals can adopt several strategies. They might implement a robust cross-validation framework, which systematically verifies the model's ability to generalize its predictions to new, unseen patient data. Additionally, integrating domain knowledge is crucial; it allows for the selection of features with established relevance to conditions like diabetes, thereby enhancing the model's predictive accuracy. Regularization techniques are also useful, as they penalize the model for complexity, effectively reducing the risk of mistaking random noise within the data for significant patterns. Moreover, training the model on a diverse and extensive set of patient data ensures that it captures the true variability of the patient population, further preventing overfitting. Lastly, before such a model is applied in a clinical environment, it's imperative to conduct clinical trials or studies that validate the model's predictions against actual patient outcomes, thereby ensuring its reliability and effectiveness in a real-world setting.

Differences in data quality

Differences in data quality refer to variations or inconsistencies in the quality of data used to create the AI model. This includes data errors, noise, or inconsistencies in data annotation. These differences can significantly impact the generalizability and reliability of AI models. When the training data contains inaccuracies, noise, or inconsistencies, it can hinder the ability of the model to make accurate predictions on new, unseen data.[5]

As an example, consider a scenario where an AI model is trained to classify images of cats and dogs. If the training data contains mislabeled images where some dogs are labeled as cats or vice versa, it introduces errors and inconsistencies in the data. As a result, the AI model may learn incorrect associations between features and labels, leading to inaccurate predictions. When tested on new, unseen images, the model's performance may be compromised due to inconsistencies in the training data.

Similarly, data quality issues can arise from *noisy data*, where irrelevant or erroneous information is present in the training dataset. This noise can mislead the model and prevent it from capturing the true underlying patterns. For example, consider the scenario where a healthcare practitioner wants to analyze patient sentiment from surveys to understand their satisfaction with a particular medical procedure. If the sentiment analysis model is trained on a dataset that includes noisy patient reviews, such as reviews with exaggerated negative experiences or unrelated comments, the model may not accurately identify the true sentiment of future patient feedback. This can lead to misleading insights and impact the healthcare practitioner's ability to make informed decisions based on patient sentiment. Inconsistencies in data annotation, such as inconsistent labeling conventions or varying levels of granularity in annotations, can also affect data quality. If different annotators have different interpretations or standards when labeling data, it can introduce inconsistencies that impact the performance and generalizability of the AI model.

Lack of standardization

The lack of standardization in healthcare data contributes to the limited generalizability of AI models.[5] Health professionals working across multiple healthcare systems may encounter challenges in integrating AI models into their practice due to the lack of standardization in data formats and interoperability. For example, if one healthcare system uses a proprietary data format for medical imaging, while another system follows a different standard, it can hinder the seamless exchange of data required for training and deploying AI models across these systems.

Lack of standardization can be caused by inconsistent data formats, variable data quality, and interoperability issues. The absence of standardized protocols for data collection, storage, and sharing poses challenges in leveraging AI effectively. Standardization efforts are necessary to harmonize data collection practices, ensure data quality, and enable interoperability, ultimately improving the generalizability of AI models across diverse healthcare settings. Health professionals can advocate for and participate in standardization initiatives to promote the use of consistent data formats and data-sharing protocols, facilitating the widespread implementation of AI in medicine.

Addressing these causes of limited generalizability requires careful consideration of dataset diversity, standardization of data collection protocols, awareness of biases in the training data, regular evaluation of model performance across different contexts, and techniques to mitigate overfitting. By addressing these factors, the generalizability of medical AI models can be improved, leading to more reliable and equitable healthcare outcomes.

Solutions to enhance generalizability

To enhance the generalizability of medical AI systems, several solutions can be implemented. These solutions focus on optimizing the design, development, and deployment of AI models in a manner that accounts for the unique challenges and requirements of the healthcare domain. By adopting these solutions, health professionals can maximize the benefits of AI while minimizing its limitations and potential risks.

Representative training data

Collecting diverse and representative datasets is crucial to improve the generalizability of AI models. Efforts should be made to include data from different demographic groups, geographical regions, and healthcare settings to reduce biases and increase inclusivity. The training data should encompass a wide range of medical conditions, patient characteristics, and treatment outcomes. By incorporating diverse data, AI models can learn from a comprehensive representation of real-world scenarios, leading to improved generalizability.

Looking at how expanded training data is used in diagnostic imaging may be helpful. AI models that are trained on diverse datasets from different imaging modalities, equipment, and patient populations can enhance generalizability in diagnostic imaging tasks. For example, AI algorithms for CT image reconstruction can benefit from training on diverse patient positioning and imaging scenarios, leading to improved precision and quality of diagnostic images.

Another example of representative training models are foundation models. Foundation models are the latest generation of AI models. A foundation model is a large machine learning model trained on massive, unlabeled, and diverse data sets. This allows them to learn general patterns and representations that can be applied to a wide range of downstream tasks. A foundation model serves as a base upon which more specialized AI applications can be built. These models have been applied to tasks such as question answering, image description, and video game playing, demonstrating their versatility and generalizability. By training AI models on diverse datasets, they can learn from a wide range of examples and contexts, enhancing their ability to generalize to new situations.

Developing large and diverse datasets is difficult, time-consuming, and expensive. A solution to this dilemma is synthetic data generation. By creating synthetic data that mimics the characteristics of real patient populations, AI models can be trained on a broader range of scenarios and variations, leading to improved generalizability. Synthetic data can help address limitations in data availability and privacy concerns while still providing realistic training samples.

Standardization and interoperability

Standardizing data formats, protocols, and interoperability frameworks is crucial for enhancing the generalizability of AI models. Standardization efforts enable seamless integration and exchange of data across different healthcare systems and institutions. This allows AI models to be trained and validated on diverse datasets from various sources, leading to more robust and generalizable performance.

In critical care, the Multiparameter Intelligent Monitoring in Intensive Care (MIMIC) datasets are one such standardized dataset.[6] MIMIC-III is a large, freely-available database comprising de-identified health data associated with over forty thousand patients who stayed in critical care units of the Beth Israel Deaconess Medical Center between 2001 and 2012. By providing a standardized, multi-parameter dataset encompassing thousands of critical care patients, MIMIC-III represents an invaluable resource for training AI algorithms that can potentially generalize well across diverse critical care populations and settings. The availability of such a large-scale benchmark dataset helps enable the creation of reproducible AI models in the critical care domain.

Continual model monitoring and updating

AI models should be continually monitored and updated to ensure their long-term performance and generalizability.[7] As healthcare environments and practices evolve, AI models need to adapt to new challenges and remain effective. Models can succumb to "data drift." Data drift refers to the phenomenon where the statistical properties of the data used by an AI model change over time, leading to declines in model performance. This can occur because of changes demographic characteristics of the patient population, changes in the way that data is recorded, or changes in the definitions or meanings of labels evolve. Said another way, "data drift" is the decline in a model's ability to make accurate predictions due to changes in the environment in which it is being used. Data drift results in the model making increasingly inaccurate predictions on new data that has different statistical properties compared to the original training data. Regular model evaluation, validation, and fine-tuning are essential to maintain their accuracy and generalizability.

Addressing bias

Mitigating bias in data collection and preprocessing is essential.[2] Careful consideration should be given to ensure fairness and equity in the representation of all population groups, minimizing the risk of biased predictions. Several techniques can help mitigate biases during the critical data collection and preprocessing phases when developing AI models. These include thoughtfully selecting data elements to avoid redundancies or irrelevant variables, continuously interrogating derived data components for hidden correlations or confounders, actively assessing and accounting for potential biases from factors like race or age group, using ensemble learning to integrate diverse modeling approaches and data sources, ensuring developer teams are inclusive and multi-disciplinary, and extensively validating the model on varied external populations to surface biases before deployment. By carefully curating the data, continuously evaluating for bias, bringing diverse perspectives, and testing performance inclusively, developers can proactively mitigate many biases that would limit the fairness, equitability, and generalizability of AI systems. Multifaceted bias mitigation must be a priority throughout the AI development pipeline.

Incorporating feedback loops

Continuous, bidirectional, feedback loops between healthcare professionals and AI system developers are crucial for improving generalizability.[1] By gathering insights and feedback from healthcare professionals who use AI systems in their practice, developers can identify areas of improvement and refine the models accordingly. This iterative process ensures that AI models become more effective and applicable to real-world healthcare scenarios. That is, they result in improved patient outcomes rather than just being optimized to performance metrics.

Updating AI algorithms

Another solution involves the continual monitoring and updating of AI algorithms.[7] AI models are sensitive to changes in the environment and may experience performance decay over time (e.g., Data Drift). The issue of performance decay has implications when it comes to regulatory approval of AI systems. The AI system approved on year one will not necessarily meet the same quality benchmarks at year two or three. Establishing dedicated units, such as AI-QI (AI quality improvement) units, within healthcare organizations can enable ongoing monitoring and maintenance of AI algorithms. These units can leverage existing quality assurance and improvement methodologies to ensure the long-term safety, effectiveness, and generalizability of AI models.

Collaboration

Additionally, collaboration between computer scientists and healthcare professionals is essential.[1] By fostering interdisciplinary collaboration, AI models can benefit from the domain expertise of healthcare professionals, ensuring that they are aligned with clinical needs and workflows. Similarly, healthcare professionals can gain a deeper understanding of AI technologies, enabling them to effectively integrate these tools into their practice and make informed decisions about their applicability.

Transfer learning

Transfer learning is a powerful technique in AI that involves taking a model that has been pre-trained on one task (e.g., Foundation model) and reusing it for a related target task.[8] It leverages knowledge from large-scale benchmark datasets to adapt AI models, enhancing their generalizability. For healthcare professionals, this means they can take advantage of existing expertise and knowledge captured in pre-trained models to address specific healthcare challenges. This is especially helpful where training data is limited.

One example is the application of transfer learning in medical image analysis. Medical imaging plays a crucial role in diagnostics and treatment planning. Deep learning models trained on large-scale datasets, such as ImageNet, have learned general image representation and feature extraction capabilities.[9] Healthcare professionals can utilize these pre-trained models and fine-tune them using medical image datasets specific to their domain, such as radiology or pathology. By fine-tuning the pre-trained models on the target medical imaging task, such as tumor detection or classification, healthcare professionals can benefit from the pre-learned features and adapt them to the specific nuances and characteristics of medical images in their domain. This approach reduces the need for large amounts of labeled medical image data and expedites the development of accurate and effective AI models for medical image analysis.

Multi-site collaborations

By pooling diverse datasets from multiple sites, AI models can be trained on a broader range of patient populations and healthcare environments, leading to improved generalization across different settings.[6,10,11] This collaborative approach benefits healthcare professionals in several ways.

One relevant example is the establishment of multi-site collaborations for research purposes. Suppose multiple hospitals or healthcare organizations join forces to create a shared database of patient records, including medical images, electronic health records, and clinical data. By combining these datasets, researchers and AI experts can develop more comprehensive and accurate AI models. For instance, if the collaboration involves hospitals from different regions or countries, it allows the inclusion of diverse patient populations, ethnicities, and healthcare practices. This diversity enhances the model's ability to generalize and adapt to various demographic and cultural contexts, improving the overall quality and applicability of the AI system in different healthcare settings.

Conclusion

The limitations of generalizability in medical AI models pose significant challenges that need to be addressed to ensure their effective and safe implementation in healthcare. Healthcare professionals must recognize that the performance and generalizability of AI models may vary across different healthcare settings, patient populations, and evolving clinical practices. These limitations stem from factors such as variations in data distributions, healthcare protocols, and contextual differences.

To overcome these limitations, several solutions can be implemented. First, robust external validation using independent datasets from diverse healthcare sites is essential to evaluate and establish the generalizability of AI models. Cross-site validation helps identify potential biases and performance variations, ensuring that models perform consistently across different institutions. Furthermore, the use of appropriate evaluation metrics, such as AUROC, precision, recall, and specificity, enables a comprehensive assessment of AI model performance in real-world scenarios.

Additionally, collaborations between researchers, clinicians, and data scientists are crucial to address the limitations of generalizability. Such collaborations can foster the development of models that are specifically designed to adapt to different healthcare settings while maintaining high performance and accuracy. Moreover, continuous monitoring and iterative improvement of AI models in real-world clinical practice can help refine their generalizability and address limitations as they arise.

Healthcare professionals need to approach the implementation and utilization of medical AI models with a critical mindset and consider the specific context and limitations of the models. While AI has the potential to revolutionize healthcare, ensuring generalizability and reliability remains a paramount concern. By acknowledging and actively addressing the limitations of generalizability, healthcare professionals can harness the full potential of AI models while providing safe and effective patient care.

References

1. Kelly CJ, Karthikesalingam A, Suleyman M, *et al.* (2019) Key challenges for delivering clinical impact with artificial intelligence. *BMC Medicine*, **17**, 195.
2. Gianfrancesco MA, Tamang S, Yazdany J, Schmajuk G. (2018) Potential biases in machine learning algorithms using Electronic Health Record data. *JAMA Internal Medicine*, **178**(11), 1544–1547.
3. Park SH, Han K. (2018) Methodologic guide for evaluating clinical performance and effect of artificial intelligence technology for medical diagnosis and prediction. Radiology, **286**(3), 800–809.
4. Christodoulou E, Ma J, Collins GS, Steyerberg EW, Verbakel JY, Van Calster B. (2019) A systematic review shows no performance benefit of machine learning over logistic regression for clinical prediction models. *Journal of Clinical Epidemiology*, **110**, 12–22.
5. Razzak MI, Naz S, Zaib A. (2017) Deep learning for medical image processing: overview, challenges and the future. In *Classification in BioApps*, Dey N, Ashour A, Borra S (eds.), Springer, Cham.
6. Johnson A, Pollard T, Shen L, *et al.* (2016) MIMIC-III, a freely accessible critical care database. *Scientific Data*, **3**, 160035 (2016).
7. Norgeot B, Glicksberg BS, Trupin L, Lituiev D, Gianfrancesco M, Oskotsky B, Schmajuk G, Yazdany J, Butte AJ. (2019) Assessment of a deep learning model based on Electronic Health Record data to forecast clinical outcomes in patients with rheumatoid arthritis. *JAMA Network Open*, **2**(3), e190606.

8. Gupta P, *et al.* (2018) Transfer learning for clinical time series analysis using recurrent neural networks. https://arxiv.org/abs/1807.01705

9. Raghu M, *et al.* (2021) Do vision transformers see like convolutional neural networks? https://arxiv.org/abs/2108.08810

10. Saeed M, Lieu C, Raber G, Mark RG. (2002) MIMIC II: a massive temporal ICU patient database to support research in intelligent patient monitoring. *Computers in Cardiology*, **29**, 641–644.

11. Fleuren LM, de Bruin DP, Tonutti M, Lalisang RCA, Elbers PWG, Gommers D, *et al.* (2021) Large-scale ICU data sharing for global collaboration: the first 1633 critically ill COVID-19 patients in the Dutch Data Warehouse. *Intensive Care Medicine*, **47**, 478–481.

Chapter 7

Explainable AI and Interpretability in Medical AI Models

What are explainability and interpretability in AI models?

AI-driven systems, such as deep learning and machine learning models, have demonstrated superior performance in various medical tasks. However, they often operate as black boxes, lacking transparency in their decision-making process. This opaqueness often leads to distrust among users, and it conflicts with our innate desire to seek meaning and understanding.[1] Further, it has raised concerns about the trustworthiness of these models and the likelihood of them being adopted. Explainability and interpretability are ways to increase understanding and trust in AI models.[1,2] They are two related but distinct concepts.

Explainability

Explainability refers to the ability to provide transparent and understandable explanations for the decisions or predictions made by these models. It addresses the need to bridge the gap between the complex inner workings of AI algorithms and the need for human interpretability and comprehension in the medical domain. Explainability in AI models is not just a problem for computer scientists, it has medical, legal, ethical, and societal implications.

From a medical standpoint, explainability enables healthcare professionals to understand how AI models arrive at their conclusions, fostering trust and allowing for validation of the decisions made by these systems. Explainability provides a transparent decision-making process where physicians and patients can understand the rationale behind treatment choices. It helps physicians and clinicians identify potential errors, biases, or limitations in the model's reasoning process, thereby ensuring patient safety and effective healthcare delivery.

From a legal perspective, explainability is crucial for addressing liability and accountability in medical AI. When AI models are involved in medical decision-making, it becomes necessary to determine responsibility for adverse outcomes or errors. Explainability allows legal professionals to assess the reasoning behind AI-generated recommendations, ensuring compliance with legal standards and regulations.

Ethically, explainability is of paramount importance in AI-driven healthcare. It promotes transparency and accountability in decision-making processes, ensuring that AI models adhere to ethical principles such as fairness, justice, and non-maleficence. Ethical evaluation involves considerations of patient autonomy, privacy, and potential biases in training data.

On a societal level, the deployment of medical AI models has broader implications. It can impact public trust in healthcare systems, influence healthcare disparities, and raise concerns about the automation of tasks traditionally performed by healthcare professionals and worker displacement. Explainability plays a vital role in addressing these societal considerations, helping stakeholders navigate the implications of AI in healthcare.

Interpretability

Interpretability primarily focuses on understanding the inner workings of the AI model, to comprehend how it generates predictions. Interpretability specifically addresses how AI models generate predictions or decisions. It involves observing the model's weights, features, and mechanisms to gain insights into its behavior and the factors that contribute to its outputs. In other words, interpretability focuses on understanding the relationship between inputs, model components, and outputs.

As an example, consider a hospital that uses an AI model to predict the likelihood of readmission for patients with a certain medical condition, such as heart failure. Interpretability in this scenario would involve examining the features and parameters of the AI model to understand which factors contribute the most to the model's predictions (e.g., age, smoking history, and salt intake). Explainability relates to the ability of an AI model to provide justifications or reasons for its predictions or decisions. It focuses on understanding the rationale behind the model's outputs by considering the significance and contribution of different variables or features within the model. Explainability involves determining why the model arrived at a particular prediction or decision by examining the parameters and hidden layers in the model. While interpretability focuses on understanding the internal mechanics of the model, explainability delves into the reasoning behind the model's specific outputs. See Table 1 for a further explanation of the differences between these two terms.

Table 1.   Explainability versus Interpretability

	Explainability	**Interpretability**
Definition	The ability to provide transparent and understandable explanations for the decisions or predictions made by AI models.	Understanding the inner workings of the AI model and how it generates predictions.
Focus	Focuses on bridging the gap between the complex inner workings of AI algorithms and the need for human interpretability and comprehension.	Focuses on understanding the relationship between inputs, model components, and outputs.
Decision-making process	Provides justifications or reasons for the model's predictions or decisions.	Observes the model's weights, features, and mechanisms to gain insights into its behavior and the factors that contribute to its outputs.

(Continued)

Table 1.   *(Continued)*

	Explainability	Interpretability
Transparency	Offers full transparency by showing the inner mechanics and decision-making process of the AI model.	Provides a general understanding of the model's behavior without revealing all the intricate details.
Target audience	Addresses the need for transparency and understanding among various stakeholders, including healthcare professionals, legal professionals, and society.	Helps professionals gain insights into the model's decisions and navigate through the data-driven insights without requiring full transparency.
Impact on performance	Often comes at the cost of performance, as the model may sacrifice accuracy or efficiency to provide detailed explanations.	Strikes a balance between performance and understanding, allowing professionals to trust the model's decisions while not having access to all the intricate details.
Use cases	Enables healthcare professionals to understand how AI models arrive at their conclusions, fostering trust and allowing for validation of the decisions made by these systems.	Helps professionals gain insights into the factors that contribute to the model's predictions, such as age, smoking history, and salt intake.
Legal and ethical considerations	Crucial for addressing liability and accountability in medical AI, ensuring compliance with legal standards and regulations.	Promotes transparency and accountability in decision-making processes, ensuring adherence to ethical principles and avoiding potential biases in training data.
Societal implications	Impacts public trust in healthcare systems, influences healthcare disparities, and raises concerns about the automation of tasks traditionally performed by healthcare professionals.	Addresses societal considerations related to AI in healthcare, helping stakeholders navigate the implications and ethical concerns of AI models.

Importance of explainability and interpretability in AI models

Explainability and interpretability are decisive issues when it comes to AI models in medicine. These concepts refer to the ability to understand and explain how AI algorithms make decisions or predictions. In the context of healthcare, where the stakes are high, and decisions directly impact patient well-being, explainability and interpretability become even more critical. Here are the key reasons why these are important in AI models in medicine:

Trust and acceptance

Explainable AI models enhance trust and acceptance among healthcare professionals, patients, and regulatory bodies. When physicians and other healthcare providers can understand and interpret the reasoning behind AI-generated recommendations or predictions, they are more likely to trust and rely on the system. Similarly, patients feel more comfortable when the decisions made by AI models can be explained to them.

Ethical and legal considerations

Explainability and interpretability play a vital role in addressing ethical and legal concerns related to AI in medicine. Healthcare professionals have a responsibility to ensure that AI algorithms are fair, unbiased, and comply with legal and regulatory standards. By having transparent and interpretable AI models, it becomes easier to identify and address potential biases, discrimination, or other ethical dilemmas that may arise.

Accountability and responsibility

In healthcare, it is essential to attribute responsibility for decisions made by AI models. If an AI algorithm makes an incorrect or harmful decision, it is crucial to understand why and who should be held accountable. Explainable and interpretable models enable thorough post-hoc analysis and facilitate the identification of any errors, biases, or limitations in the system, ensuring accountability for the outcomes.[3]

Clinical decision support and collaboration

Explainability and interpretability enhance the collaboration between AI systems and healthcare professionals. When physicians can understand how an AI model arrived at a particular recommendation, they can critically evaluate and integrate that information with their clinical expertise. This collaboration between AI and healthcare professionals leads to more effective clinical decision-making, where the strengths and limitations of both humans and machines are leveraged.

Regulatory compliance

Regulatory bodies, such as the Food and Drug Administration (FDA) in the U.S., require explainability and interpretability of AI models in healthcare.[4] These regulations would enable the FDA and manufacturers to evaluate and monitor a software product from its premarket development to post market performance. Meeting regulatory standards often involves providing evidence of the safety, effectiveness, and reliability of AI systems. Explainable models enable regulators to evaluate the algorithm's behavior, assess potential risks, and ensure compliance with existing regulations.

Education and continuous learning

Explainable and interpretable AI models also serve an educational purpose. Healthcare professionals can learn from AI systems by understanding how they arrive at certain decisions.[5] By examining the underlying reasoning and patterns used by AI models, physicians can gain insights and improve their own diagnostic and treatment skills.

Methods for explaining and interpreting AI-based medical decisions

Explaining and interpreting AI-based medical decisions is a vital step when ensuring transparency and understanding in healthcare. In this section, some methods commonly used for explaining and interpreting AI-based medical decisions are provided, along with definitions of relevant terms and examples to increase clarity.

Feature importance

Feature importance refers to the assessment of the contribution of different variables or factors in an AI model's decision-making process. It helps identify which input features have the most significant influence on the model's predictions. For example, in a machine learning model predicting the risk of heart disease, feature importance analysis may reveal that age, blood pressure, and cholesterol levels are the most critical factors driving the predictions. This information can assist healthcare professionals in understanding why a particular decision was made and help identify potential biases or confounding factors.

Rule-based explanations

Rule-based explanations involve extracting human-readable rules or decision criteria from AI models. These rules explain how the model reaches its predictions by using logical conditions and thresholds. To illustrate, a rule-based explanation for a diagnostic AI model could be: "If the patient's temperature is above 38°C, and they have a cough and shortness of breath, predict positive for COVID-19." Rule-based explanations make the decision process more transparent and allow clinicians to validate the model's decisions against their expertise.

Model visualization

The term "model visualization" refers to techniques that generate graphical representations to explain how an AI model works internally. Key goals of model visualization include depicting the overall structure of the model architecture, projecting the high-dimensional feature representations within the model down to lower dimensions that can be visualized, highlighting which parts of the input data most strongly influence the predictions, enabling interactive visuals where users can alter inputs and immediately see the impact on outputs, and analyzing model behavior across datasets to audit for desirable or problematic patterns. Overall, model visualization aims to open the "black box" of AI systems by creating human-interpretable graphics and visuals that provide insights into the model's internal mechanics, representations, and decision-making processes. By moving beyond the raw inputs and outputs of a model to visualize how information flows through the internals, model visualization techniques allow users to develop an intuitive understanding of model functions rather than treating the system as an impenetrable black box. Visual explanations enhance interpretability.[6] To give you an idea, visualizing a deep learning model's convolutional layer can reveal how it recognizes different features or patterns in medical images such as tumors or anomalies.

Local explanations

Local explanations focus on providing interpretable insights into specific predictions made by an AI model. Instead of explaining the entire model's behavior, local explanations provide information about a single prediction. One widely used method for local explanations is Local Interpretable Model-Agnostic Explanations (LIME).[7] LIME generates an explanation by approximating the model's behavior locally around the prediction of interest. For instance, LIME can highlight the specific regions in an image that influenced the AI model's diagnosis.

Counterfactual explanations

A counterfactual explanation in an AI model refers to a post-hoc explanation technique that explores the changes in the input features of the model to understand how those changes would lead to a different output or outcome.[8] It aims to answer questions such as "What would have happened if the input had been different?" or "What changes to the input would result in a desired output?" For example, consider a healthcare provider using an AI model to predict the risk of heart disease in patients.

The model utilizes various input features such as age, blood pressure, cholesterol level, and smoking status to make predictions. A healthcare provider could ask the model what changes in the patient's risk factors would have resulted in a different prediction. By altering the values of these features, such as reducing blood pressure or quitting smoking, the healthcare provider can understand the impact of these modifications on the predicted risk of heart disease. This information enables them to identify specific changes that need to be made to achieve a desired outcome, such as lowering the patient's risk level and improving their cardiovascular health. Additionally, counterfactual explanations are selective and efficient. They focus on only a limited number of important features. By providing new information about a limited number of influential features, these explanations are informative and facilitate creative problem-solving. In healthcare, this can aid physicians in devising alternative treatment plans or identifying specific risk factors that can be modified. Lastly, counterfactual explanations shed light on the decision-making process of AI medical models. They enable organizations to assess if bias is present and ensure compliance with legal regulations. For instance, if a model suggests a particular treatment option, a counterfactual explanation can help identify whether the decision was influenced by biased training data or other factors.

Certainty and confidence measures

Certainty and confidence measures indicate the level of certainty or confidence that an AI model has in its predictions.[9] Confidence is a measure of how sure an AI model is about its prediction, often expressed as a probability score, and it acknowledges the possibility of uncertainty. In contrast, certainty signifies absolute belief in the accuracy of a prediction without room for doubt. The choice between these terms depends on the nature of the AI model and the level of uncertainty it deals with. These measures provide an estimate of the model's reliability and can be used to gauge the level of trust placed in its decisions. For instance, a model might output a probability score of 0.85 for a particular diagnosis, indicating a high level of confidence in that prediction. It is important to note that these methods are not mutually exclusive and can be used in combination to provide a comprehensive understanding of AI-based medical decisions. By employing these methods, healthcare professionals can gain insights into the decision-making process of AI models, validate their predictions, identify potential biases or limitations, and ultimately build trust in the technology.

Balancing accuracy and interpretability in AI models

When it comes to AI models, finding the right balance between accuracy and interpretability is imperative.[10] This balance depends on the specific clinical context and the level of interpretability required.[11] In some cases, high accuracy might be the primary goal, while in others, interpretability might be equally important. Understanding the specific requirements of the use case is essential as it guides the balance between accuracy and interpretability. Some important considerations in this balancing act include:

Contextualize the use case

Explainable AI techniques should be designed specifically based on the targeted real-world use case and context rather than abstractly evaluating different explanation methods. This user-centered design process would start by thoroughly understanding the intended users, their background knowledge, goals, and workflows so that the explanations can be customized to align with how those users best understand complex concepts. The process should also clearly define the rationale upfront for requiring explainability in the given context, whether it be justifying recommendations, revealing biases, or educating users, as that guides the information content and evaluation methodology. Additionally, the representation of the explanations should suit the users. For instance, clinicians may prefer visual explanatory aids over pure text descriptions. Utility and efficacy should be evaluated with user studies in the intended context to ensure the explanations positively impact real-world goals and workflows. Finally, an iterative design approach should refine the explanations based on feedback from representative users. Overall, the specific clinical or practical use case context should drive explainable AI design choices, not just abstract assessment of different explanation techniques, to balance accuracy and interpretability based on the requirements and produce AI systems with meaningful real-world utility.

Select appropriate models

Different AI models offer varying degrees of interpretability. For instance, rule-based models or decision trees tend to be highly interpretable, while deep learning models can provide higher accuracy but lower interpretability. Choosing a model that strikes an appropriate balance is crucial.

Model complexity

Complex models often achieve higher accuracy but can be less interpretable.[12] Simplifying the model architecture or incorporating post-hoc interpretability techniques can help strike a balance. Techniques such as feature importance analysis, model visualization, or generating rule-based explanations can enhance interpretability without significantly sacrificing accuracy.

Collaborative approach

A collaborative approach requires engagement in interdisciplinary collaborations between healthcare professionals and data scientists. By involving clinicians in the development and validation of AI models, it is possible to ensure that both accuracy and interpretability are addressed effectively.[13]

Continuous evaluation and improvement

The performance of AI models in real-world clinical settings require regular evaluation and improvement. This can be done by gathering feedback from clinicians and patients to identify areas for improvement in both accuracy and interpretability. This iterative process helps refine the models over time.

Striking the right balance between accuracy and interpretability depends on the specific clinical scenario and the requirements of healthcare professionals. By considering the context, selecting appropriate models, simplifying complexity when necessary, promoting interdisciplinary collaboration, and continuously evaluating and improving the models, it becomes possible to achieve an optimal equilibrium between accuracy and interpretability in AI programs used in clinical practice. The following are two case studies demonstrating the benefits of interpretability of AI models in clinical medicine:

Case Study 1: Predicting diabetic retinopathy

Diabetic retinopathy is a leading cause of blindness and early detection is crucial for effective treatment. In a case study conducted by researchers at Google, an interpretable AI model was developed to predict the risk of diabetic retinopathy using retinal images.[14] The model provided a risk score, then used a technique called Gradient-weighted Class Activation Mapping (Grad-CAM) to highlight the regions of the image that contributed the most to the model's prediction. This interpretability feature allowed ophthalmologists to understand which areas of the retina influenced the AI model's decision, enabling them to validate and refine the predictions. By examining the specific regions identified by the AI model, clinicians could gain insights into the features associated with diabetic retinopathy and improve their diagnostic accuracy.

Case Study 2: Interpretable AI for early detection of lung cancer

In a study published in Nature Medicine, researchers developed an AI model to detect lung cancer from computed tomography (CT) scans.[15] The model determined whether there were signs of cancer in the image. They found that the AI model outperformed the radiologists in cases where there was no prior imaging but was on par with them when prior CT scans were available. Then, to ensure interpretability, the researchers used an approach called an attention mechanism, which highlighted the regions in the CT scans that contributed the most to the model's decision. By visualizing the areas of interest, radiologists could understand the features and patterns that the AI model relied on for its predictions. This interpretability allowed radiologists to look at those specific areas in the image to validate the AI model's findings and gain insights into the specific characteristics of lung cancer nodules, improving their confidence in the diagnostic process. Furthermore, by understanding the AI model's decision-making process, radiologists could provide more comprehensive reports and communicate the findings effectively to other healthcare professionals and patients.

These case studies demonstrate how interpretability in AI models can provide insights into the decision-making process and enhance the collaboration between AI algorithms and healthcare professionals. By visualizing and explaining the AI model's reasoning, clinicians can validate the predictions, gain knowledge about disease characteristics, and refine their diagnostic and treatment approaches. Interpretability promotes transparency, trust, and accountability, leading to more effective integration of AI technology into clinical practice.

Conclusion

This chapter on explainability and interpretability in medical AI models emphasizes the critical importance of transparency and understandability in the decision-making process of AI systems. The adoption of AI models in healthcare settings poses challenges due to the high stakes involved and the need to ensure patient safety. While AI algorithms may outperform humans in certain tasks, the lack of explainability hinders their widespread acceptance and trust. It is crucial to address the black-box nature of AI models and provide meaningful explanations for their predictions and recommendations.

Efforts should be directed towards achieving adequate human-AI teaming performance, where human users can comprehend and trust the decisions made by AI systems. Human-centered design principles should be employed to guide the development of explainable medical AI tools, considering the needs and perspectives of clinical stakeholders and patients. Guidelines and evidence from systematic reviews emphasize the importance of designing trustworthy AI systems that align with human decision-making processes and improve patient outcomes. To build trust and confidence in medical AI, explainability must be prioritized. AI algorithms used for diagnosis and prognosis should not rely on black-box approaches, and efforts should be made to develop interpretable models that provide meaningful explanations for their decisions. While technological challenges exist, research in explainable AI has been reignited to address these issues.

The multidisciplinary nature of explainability in medical AI necessitates collaboration among technologists, legal experts, medical professionals, and patients. Ethical evaluations should be conducted, considering principles such as autonomy, beneficence, nonmaleficence, and justice. Adequate explanations can enhance accountability, regulation, and the adoption of AI-driven tools in clinical practice.

References

1. Tonekaboni S, *et al.* (2019) What clinicians want: contextualizing explainable machine learning for clinical end use. https://arxiv.org/abs/1905.05134
2. Holzinger A, Langs G, Denk H, Zatloukal K, Müller H. (2019) Causability and explainability of artificial intelligence in medicine. *WIREs Data Mining and Knowledge Discovery*, **9**(4), e1312. https://doi.org/10.1002/widm.1312
3. Lamy JB, Sekar B, Guezennec G, Bouaud J, Séroussi B. (2019) Explainable artificial intelligence for breast cancer: a visual case-based reasoning approach. *Artificial Intelligence in Medicine*, **94**, 42–53.
4. (2021) Artificial intelligence and machine learning in software as a medical device. https://www.fda.gov/medical-devices/software-medical-device-samd/artificial-intelligence-and-machine-learning-software-medical-device
5. Shortliffe EH, Sepúlveda MJ. (2018) Clinical decision support in the era of artificial intelligence. *JAMA Network*, **320**(21), 2199–2200.
6. Hohman F, *et al.* (2019) GAMUT: a design probe to understanding how data scientists understand machine learning models. In *Proceedings of the 2019 CHI Conference on Human Factors in Computing Systems (CHI '19)*, Association for Computing Machinery, New York, USA, Paper 579, 1–13.

7. Ribeiro, Marco Tulio, Sameer Singh, Carlos Guestrin. (2016) "Why should i trust you?: Explaining the predictions of any classifier." In *Proceedings of the 22nd ACM SIGKDD International Conference on Knowledge Discovery and Data Mining (KDD '16)*. Association for Computing Machinery, New York, USA, 1135–1144.

8. Wachter S, Mittelstadt B, Russell C. (2017) Counterfactual explanations without opening the black box: Automated decisions and the GDPR. *Harvard Journal of Law & Technology*, **31**(2).

9. Gilpin LH, Bau D, Yuan BZ, Bajwa A, Specter M, Kagal L. (2018) Explaining explanations: an overview of interpretability of machine learning. In *2018 IEEE 5th International Conference on Data Science and Advanced Analytics (DSAA)*, Turin, Italy, 80–89.

10. Bell A, Solano-Kamiko I, *et al.* (2022) It's just not that simple: an empirical study of the accuracy-explainability trade-off in machine learning for public policy. In *Proceedings of the 2022 ACM Conference on Fairness, Accountability, and Transparency (FAccT '22)*. Association for Computing Machinery, New York, USA, 248–266.

11. van der Veer SN, *et al.* (2021) Trading off accuracy and explainability in AI decision-making: findings from 2 citizens' juries. *Journal of the American Medical Informatics Association*, **28**(10), 2128–2138.

12. Linardatos P, Papastefanopoulos V, Kotsiantis S. (2020) Explainable AI: a review of machine learning interpretability methods. *Entropy*, **23**(1), 18.

13. Kelly CJ, Karthikesalingam A, Suleyman M, *et al.* (2019) Key challenges for delivering clinical impact with artificial intelligence. *BMC Medicine*, **17**, 195.

14. Diagnosing diabetic retinopathy with AI. https://about.google/intl/ALL_us/stories/seeingpotential/

15. Ardila D, Kiraly AP, Bharadwaj S, *et al.* (2019) End-to-end lung cancer screening with three-dimensional deep learning on low-dose chest computed tomography. *Nature Medicine*, **25**, 954–961.

Chapter 8

Ethical Implications of AI in Medicine

Introduction

In the rapidly evolving landscape of healthcare, the integration of artificial intelligence holds immense promise for transforming medical practice and improving patient outcomes. However, along with examining its potential benefits, the ethical implications of Artificial Intelligence (AI) in healthcare cannot be overlooked.

Medical ethics

Before discussing the particulars of the ethics of the use of AI technologies, it may be helpful to quickly review how physicians should address ethical dilemmas in general. Ethical frameworks in the medical setting are structured approaches that guide healthcare professionals in making ethical decisions and navigating complex moral situations.[1] They are a set of guidelines or principles designed to guide decision-making and conduct, particularly in complex or morally challenging situations. They serve as a foundational structure to help individuals, organizations, or societies determine what is right, fair, and just.

In the medical field, ethical frameworks help healthcare professionals consider various ethical principles and apply them to clinical practice. These frameworks often revolve around key ethical principles, such as beneficence (promoting patient well-being), non-maleficence (avoiding harm), autonomy (respecting patient choices and self-determination), and justice (fair distribution of resources and equal treatment).[2] They assist in balancing these principles and resolving conflicts that may arise between them. Medical ethical frameworks also address specific issues relevant to the healthcare context. For example, frameworks may provide guidance on obtaining informed consent from patients, ensuring truth-telling and confidentiality, and navigating conflicts of interest.[3] They offer a structured approach to ethical problem-solving and help healthcare professionals consider the ethical implications of their actions.

Here are key points about medical ethics and AI systems that all healthcare professionals should be aware of:

Patient autonomy and informed consent

AI applications in healthcare have the potential to influence medical decision-making. It is essential to ensure that patients remain active participants in their healthcare journey. Physicians should prioritize obtaining informed consent from patients, explaining how AI is used in their care and providing them with the opportunity to ask questions and express their preferences.[4,5]

Trust and transparency

Trust is the foundation of the physician-patient relationship.[6-8] Physicians must understand and communicate the limitations, risks, and benefits of AI systems to their patients.[9] This assumes explainability of AI model decisions. Transparency in the development, training, and validation of AI algorithms is crucial to maintain patient trust and ensure that they understand how AI-based decisions are made. Conversely, a lack of transparency in how AI systems make decisions can impede healthcare professionals' ability to understand the reasoning behind the system's conclusions and identify potential sources of error.

Avoiding bias and ensuring fairness

AI systems are only as unbiased as the data they are trained on. It is crucial that the healthcare professional understand and address potential biases in AI algorithms that could result in health disparities or unequal access to care.[10,11] Continuous auditing of AI systems can help identify and correct for bias.[12] Furthermore, diverse, and inclusive datasets should be used to train AI models to ensure fairness in healthcare outcomes.[13]

Impact on the healthcare provider-patient relationship

The introduction of AI technologies may alter the dynamics of the healthcare provider-patient relationship[14] or even dehumanize it.[15] Patients may worry that their medical information being put into an AI system is not secure.[16] They may worry that unlike their healthcare provider, the AI system may not have their best interests at heart or that the populations used to create the data sets in the AI model are not representative of the patient.[17,18] Some patients may worry about provider de-skilling caused by the AI model and lose trust in their provider's ability to make sound healthcare decisions for them.[19] Healthcare providers should be mindful of these issues and maintain empathy, compassion, and a human connection with patients while integrating AI tools into their practice. Open communication about the role of AI and the physician's expertise is vital to preserving patient trust and engagement.

Ethical decision-making

Physicians must navigate the ethical challenges associated with AI-driven healthcare. This includes considering the potential risks and benefits, ensuring patient welfare, respecting patient privacy, and upholding professional integrity. Ethical frameworks and principles such as beneficence, autonomy, and justice should guide decision-making in AI-enabled medical practice.

Incorporating ethics in AI design and implementation

Ethical considerations should be integrated into the design and implementation of AI systems.[20] Ethical guidelines and principles, such as those addressing privacy, data security, and informed consent, should be followed during the development and deployment of AI technologies in healthcare. Collaboration between physicians, computer scientists, ethicists, and regulatory bodies can help ensure ethical AI practices.

Ethical frameworks and regulatory considerations

Existing ethical frameworks, such as those developed by professional medical associations or institutions, guide ethical AI use in healthcare. Physicians should be aware of these frameworks and follow relevant legal and regulatory requirements in their jurisdiction. Compliance with privacy regulations, data protection laws, and institutional policies is crucial when using AI in a medical setting.

Data privacy and security considerations specific to AI applications in healthcare

The use of AI in healthcare requires the collection, storage, and analysis of very large amounts of patient data,[21] raising concerns about data privacy and security. In fact a Pew Research poll found that 37% of Americans felt that the use of AI in medicine would make the security of medical records worse.[18] It is crucial to implement robust measures to protect patient information and ensure compliance with privacy regulations to maintain patient trust and confidentiality.

Balancing beneficence, autonomy, and justice in AI-enabled medical decision-making

Achieving a balance between beneficence, autonomy, and justice is essential when developing AI-enabled medical decision-making models.[23,24]

Beneficence emphasizes the potential of AI systems to improve patient outcomes and resource utilization by providing evidence-based recommendations and predictive analytics. This leads to improved patient outcomes and efficient resource utilization. As an example, AI algorithms can accurately diagnose skin cancer, assisting dermatologists in delivering timely and accurate diagnoses.

Respecting patient autonomy is another key aspect of AI-enabled medical decision-making.[23,25] AI systems should provide patients with comprehensive information about their health conditions, treatment options, and potential outcomes, empowering them to make informed decisions based on personalized data-driven insights. By actively involving patients in their care, AI tools can support autonomous decision-making.

Justice plays a critical role in ensuring equitable access to AI technologies and addressing algorithmic bias. To ensure justice in AI-enabled medical decision-making, it is important to address issues of algorithmic bias and ensure equitable access to AI technologies. Algorithmic bias in the setting of AI in medicine refers to the presence of unfair or discriminatory outcomes resulting from the use of algorithms or AI systems in healthcare decision-making processes.[26] It occurs when the algorithms, due to the data they are trained on or the underlying design, exhibit preferential treatment or unfairness towards certain individuals or groups, leading to disparities in the quality of care, diagnosis, treatment, or access to healthcare services.[27] AI-enabled medical decision-making respects patient autonomy by providing patients with comprehensive information about their health conditions, treatment options, and potential outcomes. Patients can make informed decisions based on personalized data-driven insights, empowering them to actively participate in their care.

To balance beneficence, autonomy, and justice in AI-enabled medical decision-making, a comprehensive approach is needed. This involves the responsible design and development of AI systems that prioritize patient well-being, provide transparent explanations for their recommendations, and adhere to ethical principles. Additionally, ongoing monitoring, evaluation, and regulation are necessary to ensure that AI technologies promote fairness, inclusivity, and patient-centered care. In summary, achieving a balance between beneficence, autonomy, and justice in AI-enabled medical decision-making requires a holistic approach that leverages AI's potential to improve patient outcomes while respecting patient autonomy and addressing issues of bias and fairness. By upholding these principles, AI systems can support healthcare providers and patients in making well-informed, personalized decisions that prioritize patient well-being and promote equitable access to care.

Bias in AI models

There is increasing concern that AI systems might reflect and magnify existing human biases, potentially diminishing the quality of their performance in traditionally underrepresented populations like women, individuals of low socioeconomic status, or Black patients.[28,29] The implications of these biases become extremely grave in the context of underdiagnosis. This phenomenon happens when an AI system incorrectly identifies a person with a particular disease as healthy, potentially causing delays in providing appropriate medical care. This problem of bias and underdiagnosis in AI can create significant health disparities and exacerbate existing inequities,[29] calling for immediate attention and redress.

Addressing algorithmic bias

Algorithmic bias in medical AI models refers to the presence of systematic and unfair discrimination in the decision-making processes and outcomes of these models. When developing and training AI models for medical applications, biases can inadvertently be introduced due to various factors, including biased training data, flawed algorithms, or the interpretation of the results.[30] This bias can exacerbate existing inequities in healthcare, such as those related to socioeconomic status, race, ethnicity, religion, gender, disability, or sexual orientation, and impact the accuracy and fairness of the AI models' predictions and recommendations.[31,32]

The consequences of algorithmic bias in medical AI models can disproportionately affect disadvantaged populations, leading to less accurate predictions or underestimation of the need for care in these groups.[11] For example, a widely used commercial prediction algorithm, which is employed by health systems to identify and assist patients with complex health needs, exhibits significant racial bias. This algorithm predicts healthcare costs rather than the actual health status of patients. However, the algorithm's predictions result in racial bias. The bias is manifested in the fact that Black patients, with the same risk score as White patients, are found to be in worse health. This implies that Black patients are not receiving the level of care they need. The bias arises due to unequal access to healthcare services. This inequality leads to lower healthcare spending on Black patients compared to White patients, even when their health conditions are equally severe. Addressing this bias would significantly increase the percentage of Black patients receiving additional healthcare support. This underscores the importance of rectifying the bias to ensure equitable healthcare delivery.[28] To address algorithmic bias in medical AI models, various strategies and mitigation techniques have been proposed. These include:

Diverse and representative data

It is crucial to ensure that the data used to train AI algorithms is diverse, representative, and free from bias is essential.[33] This can involve collecting data from a wide range of demographics and socioeconomic backgrounds, accounting for different cultural contexts, and mitigating underrepresentation.

Fairness and bias detection

Employing fairness metrics and bias detection techniques during the development and evaluation of AI models can help identify and mitigate bias.[34] Regularly monitoring the performance of algorithms across different subpopulations can aid in detecting and addressing disparities.

Bias mitigation

Addressing bias in AI datasets involves various techniques at different stages of the AI development pipeline, from data collection and preprocessing to model training and evaluation.[35] These debiasing techniques are crucial to mitigate systematic errors that can have significant social and ethical implications, such as exacerbating disparities and perpetuating biases.

Data collection and preprocessing

The initial stage of debiasing starts from gathering and cleaning the data. This includes being aware of potential biases in the way data is collected and ensuring it represents all relevant groups equitably. For instance, data could have "sample bias" if the training dataset does not accurately represent the full scope of the population, leading to biased outputs.

Reweighing examples

During the preprocessing stage, one technique used to mitigate bias is reweighing the examples, which adjusts the weight of each instance in the training set to ensure fair representation of different groups. Imagine a dataset used for predicting the risk of heart disease. This dataset includes patient attributes like age, gender, cholesterol levels, blood pressure, and history of smoking. However, suppose the dataset has a bias: it contains more male than female patients, and historically, treatment protocols were more optimized for male physiology, leading to better outcomes for male patients in the dataset. To reweigh this example, one would give the existing female patients a higher weight and the males would be assigned a lower weight. This decreases the bias to males and makes the models output more accurate.

In-processing techniques

In-processing techniques in machine learning refer to methods applied during the training phase of a model or algorithm to improve its performance, ensure fairness, or handle specific types of data. These techniques are integral to the model training process and can directly influence how the model learns from the data. In-processing interventions are applied during the model's learning process. Techniques such as "Classification with Fairness Constraints," "Prejudice Remover Regularizer," and "Adversarial Debiasing" are used. Adversarial debiasing is a technique in machine learning aimed at reducing bias in predictive models. It is particularly relevant in the context of fair machine learning, where the goal is to ensure that models do not perpetuate or exacerbate existing biases, such as those based on race, gender, or other sensitive attributes. In adversarial debiasing, two models are built: one to predict the target based on feature engineering and preprocessing steps taken on training data and an adversary model to predict a sensitive attribute based on the predictions of the first model. Ideally, in the absence of a bias, the adversary model should not predict the sensitive attribute well.

Algorithmic de-biasing

This involves developing an algorithm to learn a specific task while understanding the structure of the training data, allowing it to identify and minimize hidden biases.[37] Different approaches can be taken to de-bias algorithms. They may include refining the data collection and processing methods to avoid perpetuating existing societal biases, creating mathematical frameworks to control the amplification of bias, or reevaluating the metrics used to measure algorithmic success.

Subgroup analysis

Subgroup analysis is an approach to decreasing bias in a data set. This technique entails dividing the data into smaller subsets, or "subgroups," based on different characteristics like age, gender, race, socioeconomic status, or any other relevant variables.[27] It can be a useful technique in mitigating bias in an AI data including accounting for variability and highlighting underrepresented groups. This strategy can significantly aid in reducing bias in AI datasets through several mechanisms:

- Better representation: By dividing the data into smaller subgroups based on unique traits, it allows for a more thorough representation of different sections of the population. This detailed approach ensures that every subgroup has a voice in the AI system, promoting equality and minimizing systemic biases.
- Uncovering hidden patterns: Often, biases arise from hidden or overlooked patterns in the data. Subgroup analysis can help uncover these patterns by focusing on specific subgroups within the larger dataset, providing a more nuanced understanding of the data.
- Exploratory analysis: Subgroup analysis can be used as an exploratory tool, helping researchers identify subsets of the population with unique or significant characteristics. This can lead to the development of more tailored and personalized AI systems.

Once specific biases have been identified through subgroup analysis, they can be effectively addressed and mitigated.

In an illustrative case, a clinical AI model was developed in 2021 at the Vector Institute in Toronto for diagnosing certain conditions using chest radiographs. Initial application of the model showed an underdiagnosis bias, particularly in underserved patient populations. This bias was attributed to differences in the performance of the AI system on different racial and ethnic groups, with the model having poorer performance on patients from certain backgrounds. To mitigate this bias, the researchers performed a subgroup analysis based on race, ethnicity, and socioeconomic status among other variables. They found that the model's performance varied significantly across these subgroups. Upon further investigation, it was identified that the data used to train the model was not adequately representative of these underserved patient populations. For this reason, the researchers incorporated more diverse data into the training set, including a larger representation of underserved patient groups, and retrained the model. They also used advanced machine learning techniques to better capture complex interactions among the variables. This revised model, when tested, showed a significant decrease in bias compared to the original model. The results of this subgroup analysis not only improved the accuracy of the model, but also provided crucial insights into the sources of bias within the AI model. This allowed the researchers to develop more equitable AI tools for clinical practice.

Though this technique can be a powerful tool for decreasing bias in algorithms, it is important to understand that it must be carefully conducted to avoid certain pitfalls such as, overfitting, "chasing noise" or making false discoveries due to random variation. It is also recommended to have a clear hypothesis for the subgroup analysis and to adjust for multiple comparisons to prevent incorrect conclusions.

Policy changes

Long-term de-biasing can be implemented through policy changes at different levels, including medical funding agencies and standards organizations, to prevent biases from being perpetuated by AI devices. Addressing bias in AI systems requires constant vigilance and active intervention at each step of the model development process. While the techniques described can mitigate bias, they may not eliminate it, highlighting the need for continued research and development in this area.

Ethical AI design

It is important to integrate ethical considerations into the design and development of AI systems. Ensuring transparency, interpretability, and explainability of AI algorithms can help identify and rectify biases. By involving interdisciplinary teams, including ethicists and domain experts, institutions can contribute to more inclusive and responsible AI design. Healthcare providers should strive for fairness and inclusivity in AI design, implementation, and access, considering diverse patient populations and their unique healthcare needs.

The role of interdisciplinary collaboration in addressing ethical challenges

Interdisciplinary collaboration is necessary to address the ethical challenges associated with AI-driven healthcare.[39] In the context of AI, collaboration among physicians, data scientists, ethicists, policymakers, and other stakeholders is essential for navigating the complex ethical landscape. By bringing together diverse expertise and perspectives, interdisciplinary teams can work toward developing comprehensive frameworks, guidelines, and policies that promote responsible AI development, deployment, and governance.

Team-based approach

Interdisciplinary collaboration among physicians, data scientists, ethicists, policymakers, and other stakeholders is essential in navigating the ethical challenges of AI-driven healthcare. Collaborative efforts can lead to comprehensive frameworks, guidelines, and policies that promote responsible AI development, deployment, and governance.

Ethical review boards

An ethical review board in the context of using AI in clinical medicine is a committee or regulatory body responsible for evaluating and overseeing the ethical considerations associated with the use of AI technologies in healthcare settings. The primary purpose of an ethical review board is to ensure that the implementation and deployment of AI systems in clinical medicine align with ethical principles, respect patient rights, and mitigate potential risks. Healthcare institutions should establish ethical review boards comprised of professionals from diverse disciplines that can ensure that AI applications in healthcare align with ethical standards. These boards can provide guidance, review research protocols, and evaluate the potential risks and benefits of AI implementation.

Ethical frameworks and regulatory considerations for AI in healthcare

AI has tremendous potential to transform healthcare but it also raises important ethical and regulatory considerations.

Overview of existing ethical frameworks for AI in healthcare

To ensure ethical AI implementation, various frameworks have been developed. The IEEE P7000 working group provides a series of guidelines for ethical considerations in AI systems.[40] These guidelines cover aspects such as transparency, accountability, and data privacy. The Belmont Report is a significant document in the field of medical ethics and research.[43] It was created by the National Commission for the Protection of Human Subjects of Biomedical and Behavioral Research in 1979. The Belmont Report provides ethical principles and guidelines for conducting research involving human subjects. Its primary focus is on protecting the rights, well-being, and autonomy of individuals participating in medical and scientific research. While the Belmont Report was not specifically focused on AI, it offers ethical principles applicable to research and healthcare, such as respect for autonomy, beneficence, and justice.[43] These frameworks emphasize the importance of ethical decision-making, avoiding bias, and protecting individuals' rights and well-being.

Legal and regulatory landscape for AI in healthcare

AI implementation in healthcare is subject to legal and regulatory requirements.[41,42] Data protection regulations, such as the General Data Protection Regulation (GDPR) in Europe, play a crucial role in safeguarding patient data and ensuring privacy. Regulatory bodies, such as the U.S. Food and Drug Administration (FDA), oversee the safety and effectiveness of AI applications in healthcare. Compliance with these regulations is essential to maintain patient trust, protect sensitive information, and uphold ethical standards.

International perspectives and guidelines for AI ethics in healthcare

International organizations and initiatives have developed guidelines to address AI ethics in healthcare. The World Health Organization (WHO) published a report on the ethics and governance of AI for health, emphasizing the need to prioritize ethics and human rights in AI design and use.[43] The report provides guidance on maximizing AI benefits while minimizing harm and promoting equitable access to AI technologies. Additionally, mapping reviews have identified ethical issues in AI healthcare applications, highlighting the importance of evidence-informed approaches and addressing gaps in ethical considerations.[44]

Ethical frameworks and regulatory considerations for AI in healthcare

Ethical frameworks and regulatory considerations are critical for the responsible deployment of AI in healthcare. Existing frameworks, such as the IEEE P7000 series[45] and the Belmont Report,[46] offer guidance on ethical decision-making. The Belmont Report provides a comprehensive framework of ethical principles and guidelines for conducting research involving human subjects. This legal and regulatory landscape, including data protection regulations and oversight by regulatory bodies like the FDA, ensure compliance and patient safety. International perspectives and guidelines, exemplified by WHO's report, stress the importance of ethics, human rights, and equitable access to AI in healthcare. By integrating these frameworks and considerations, we can promote the ethical use of AI in healthcare and maximize its potential for improving patient outcomes while protecting individual rights and ensuring transparency and accountability.

Real-world examples of ethical challenges in AI-driven healthcare

To provide concrete illustrations of ethical implications, consider the following real-world examples:

Privacy and data security

The implementation of AI technologies in healthcare raises concerns about the access, use, and control of patient data, especially when owned by private entities. The nature of the implementation of AI could mean that these corporations, hospitals, and clinics, will have a greater than typical role in obtaining, utilizing, and protecting patient health information. This raises privacy issues relating to implementation and data security. There are growing discussions and concerns regarding privacy issues relating to the implementation and data security of AI in healthcare. This is especially true after incidents in 2020, where the healthcare sector experienced many data breaches, with 41.4 million patient records breached,[47] indicating the many vulnerabilities in data security. Additionally, a 2022 analysis of hospitals' websites by journalists at "The Markup" revealed that one-third of the top 100 hospitals in the United States are sending patient data to Facebook via a tracker called Meta Pixel, without obtaining consent from patients.[48] These cases emphasize the need for robust privacy measures and data security protocols to protect patient information.

Bias and discrimination

AI algorithms can inherit biases from the data they are trained on, leading to disparities in healthcare delivery and outcomes. A 2019 study by Heidi Ledford published in the journal Nature revealed how an AI system used for triaging patients in emergency departments exhibited racial bias.[49] This AI algorithm, which is widely used in U.S. hospitals to predict which patients would benefit from extra care management, was biased against Black patients, resulting in less access to necessary care for this population. This demonstrates the importance of addressing algorithmic bias and ensuring fairness in AI models.

These examples illustrate the challenges of privacy, data security, and bias in the implementation of AI in healthcare, emphasizing the need for robust privacy measures, data security protocols, and efforts to address algorithmic bias.

Lessons learned and best practices for addressing ethical and legal implications

Addressing the ethical and legal implications of using AI in medical care requires a careful approach and the implementation of best practices. Several lessons have been learned and principles have been proposed to guide the responsible development and deployment of AI in healthcare.

Firstly, ethics and human rights should be at the heart of AI design, deployment, and use in healthcare. The World Health Organization (WHO) emphasizes the importance of placing ethics and human rights as core considerations when utilizing AI in healthcare.[43] This involves ensuring transparency, accountability, and fairness in AI systems.

Secondly, comprehensive legal and ethical frameworks are necessary to address the challenges posed by AI in healthcare. These frameworks should be developed in collaboration with various stakeholders and should consider issues such as data privacy, bias and discrimination, patient autonomy, and accountability. It is important to establish guidelines and regulations that govern the collection, storage, and use of patient data in AI-driven systems, while also safeguarding the privacy and security of individuals.

Lastly, ongoing monitoring, evaluation, and continuous learning are essential to identify and address any unintended consequences or ethical concerns that may arise during the implementation of AI in medical care.[28,48] Monitoring and evaluation also allow healthcare professionals to assess the performance and impact of AI systems in real-world clinical settings. This includes tracking factors like diagnostic accuracy, patient outcomes, and workflow efficiency. By doing so, healthcare institutions can identify any issues that may arise, such as biases in the AI algorithms or unexpected patient safety concerns. Regular assessment of AI algorithms and their impact on patient outcomes and equity is imperative. This includes addressing issues related to transparency, explainability, and algorithmic bias.

Conclusion

Key ethical and legal considerations in AI in medicine revolve around the balance between innovation and patient well-being. AI holds immense potential for improving healthcare delivery but it must be guided by ethical principles and human rights. One crucial aspect is ensuring patient privacy, data security, and informed consent to address concerns about privacy, discrimination, and psychological harm. Another key consideration is the responsible use of AI algorithms, ensuring fairness, transparency, and accountability to mitigate biases and promote trust. Additionally, maintaining the patient-provider relationship and clarifying the roles of AI systems and healthcare professionals are essential for ethical implementation. These considerations should guide policymakers, healthcare practitioners, and developers in establishing guidelines, regulations, and best practices for AI in medicine, promoting the responsible and ethical deployment of AI technologies while prioritizing patient welfare.

Ongoing ethical debates in the field of AI in medicine revolve around the transparency and explainability of AI systems. As AI algorithms become more complex and sophisticated, it becomes essential to understand how they arrive at their decisions. Ensuring transparency and interpretability of AI models is critical to building trust among healthcare professionals and patients. Furthermore, the involvement of stakeholders, including patients, healthcare providers, and AI designers, in the ethical design and application of AI systems can lead to more inclusive and patient-centered approaches.

References

1. Beauchamp TL, Childress JF. (2013) Principles of biomedical ethics (7th Edition). New York, NY: Oxford University Press, 25–26.
2. Varkey B. (2021) Principles of clinical ethics and their application to practice. *Medical Principles and Practice*, **30**(1):17–28.
3. American Medical Association. (2016) Code of medical ethics: current opinions with annotations. https://www.ama-assn.org/delivering-care/ethics/code-medical-ethics-overview
4. Esmaeilzadeh P. (2019) The effects of public concern for information privacy on the adoption of Health Information Exchanges (HIEs) by healthcare entities. *Health Communication*, **34**(10), 1202–1211.
5. Esmaeilzadeh P, Mirzaei T, Dharanikota S. (2021) Patients' perceptions toward human-artificial intelligence interaction in health care: experimental study. *Journal of Medical Internet Research*, **23**(11), e25856.
6. Beauchamp T, Childless J. (1989) Principles of Biomedical Ethics (3rd Edition). New York, NY: Oxford University Press.
7. Emanuel EJ, Dubler NN. (1995) Preserving the physician-patient relationship in the era of managed care. *JAMA Network*, **273**, 323–329.
8. Quinn TP, Senadeera M, Jacobs S, Coghlan S, Le V. (2021) Trust and medical AI: the challenges we face and the expertise needed to overcome them. *Journal of the American Medical Informatics Association*, **28**(4), 890–894.
9. Schiff D, Borenstein J. (2019) How should clinicians communicate with patients about the roles of artificially intelligent team members? *AMA Journal of Ethics*, **21**(2), E138–E145.
10. Chen Y, Clayton EW, Novak LL, Anders S, Malin B. (2023) Human-centered design to address biases in artificial intelligence. *Journal of Medical Internet Research*, **25**, e43251.
11. Norori N, Hu Q, Aellen FM, Faraci FD, Tzovara A. (2021) Addressing bias in big data and AI for health care: A call for open science. *Patterns*, **2**(10), 100347.

12. Lee NT, Rensnick P, Barton G. (2019) Algorithmic bias detection and mitigation: best practices and policies to reduce consumer harms. https://www.brookings.edu/articles/algorithmic-bias-detection-and-mitigation-best-practices-and-policies-to-reduce-consumer-harms/

13. Rajkomar A, Hardt M, Howell MD, Corrado G, Chin MH. (2018) Ensuring fairness in machine learning to advance health equity. *Annals of Internal Medicine*, **169**(12), 866–872.

14. Niel O, Bastard P. (2019) Artificial intelligence in nephrology: core concepts, clinical applications, and perspectives. *American Journal of Kidney Diseases*, **74**(6), 803–810.

15. Sparrow R, Hatherley J. (2020) High hopes for "Deep Medicine"? AI, economics, and the future of care. *Hastings Center Report*, **50**(1), 14–17.

16. Richardson JP, Smith C, Curtis S, *et al.* (2021) Patient apprehensions about the use of artificial intelligence in healthcare. *npj Digital Medicine*, **4**, 140.

17. Longoni C, Bonezzi A, Morewedge CK. (2019) Resistance to medical artificial intelligence. *Journal of Consumer Research*, **46**(4), 629–650.

18. Tyson A, *et al.* (2023) 60% of Americans would be uncomfortable with provider relying on AI in their own health care. https://www.pewresearch.org/science/2023/02/22/60-of-americans-would-be-uncomfortable-with-provider-relying-on-ai-in-their-own-health-care/

19. V. potential impact of AI on the doctor-patient relationship. https://www.coe.int/en/web/bioethics/potential-impact-of-ai-on-the-doctor-patient-relationship#{%22123746107%22:[4]}

20. Hine C, Nilforooshan R, Barnaghi P. (2022) Ethical considerations in design and implementation of home-based smart care for dementia. *Nursing Ethics*, **29**(4), 1035–1046.

21. Corea F. (2019) An introduction to data: everything you need to know about AI, big data and data science. Cham, Switzerland: Springer, 1–5.

22. Beil M, Proft I, van Heerden D, Sviri S, van Heerden PV. (2019) Ethical considerations about artificial intelligence for prognostication in intensive care. *Intensive Care Medicine Experimental*, **7**(1), 70.

23. WHO guidance. (2021) Ethics and governance of artificial intelligence for health. https://www.who.int/publications/i/item/9789240029200

24. Barry MJ, Edgman-Levitan S. (2012) Shared decision making--pinnacle of patient-centered care. N Engl J Med. **366**(9), 780–781.

25. Mittermaier M, Raza MM, Kvedar JC. (2023) Bias in AI-based models for medical applications: challenges and mitigation strategies. *npj Digital Medicine* **6**, 113.

26. Vokinger KN, Feuerriegel S, Kesselheim AS. (2021) Mitigating bias in machine learning for medicine. *Communications in Medicine*, **1**, 25.

27. Seyyed-Kalantari L, Zhang H, McDermott MBA, *et al.* (2021) Underdiagnosis bias of artificial intelligence algorithms applied to chest radiographs in under-served patient populations. *Nature Medicine*, **27**, 2176–2182. https://doi.org/10.1038/s41591-021-01595-0

28. Obermeyer Z, Powers B, Vogeli C, Mullainathan S. (2019) Dissecting racial bias in an algorithm used to manage the health of populations. *Proceedings of the National Academy of Sciences*, **116**(16), 7771–7776.

29. Panch T, Mattie H, Celi LA. (2019) The "inconvenient truth" about AI in healthcare. *Npj Digital Medicine*, **2**, 77.

30. Gijsberts CM, *et al.* (2015) Race/ethnic differences in the associations of the ramingham risk factors with carotid IMT and cardiovascular events. *PloS ONE*, **10**, e0132321.

31. Hermansson J, Kahan T. (2017) Systematic review of validity assessments of Framingham risk score results in health economic modelling of lipid-modifying therapies in Europe. *Pharmacoeconomics*, **36**, 205–213.

32. Phillips PJ, *et al.* (2021) Four principles of explainable artificial intelligence. https://nvlpubs.nist.gov/nistpubs/ir/2021/NIST.IR.8312.pdf

33. Bøttcher L, Flach P, Lykkegaard NB. (2019) Ethical machine learning–a risk-based approach. *AI Ethics*, 1-14.

34. Manyika J, Silberg J, Presten B. (2019) What do we do about the biases in AI? https://hbr.org/2019/10/what-do-we-do-about-the-biases-in-ai

35. Maddali S. (2022) How to address data bias in machine learning. https://towardsdatascience.com/how-to-address-data-bias-in-machine-learning-c6a45db53b8d

36. Conner-Simons A. (2019) An AI that "de-biases" algorithms. https://www.csail.mit.edu/news/ai-de-biases-algorithms

37. Kusters R, Misevic D, Berry H, Cully A, Le Cunff Y, Dandoy L, Díaz-Rodríguez N, Ficher M, Grizou J, Othmani A, Palpanas T, Komorowski M, Loiseau P, Moulin Frier C, Nanini S, Quercia D, Sebag M, Soulié Fogelman F, Taleb S, Tupikina L, Sahu V, Vie JJ, Wehbi F. (2020) Interdisciplinary research in artificial intelligence: challenges and opportunities. *Front Big Data*, **3**, 577974.

38. IEEE Standards Association Statement of Intention. (2018) Our role in addressing ethical considerations of Autonomous and Intelligent Systems (A/IS). https://standards.ieee.org/wp-content/uploads/import/documents/other/ethical-considerations-ai-as-29mar2018.pdf

39. Pesapane F, *et al.* (2021) Legal and regulatory framework for AI solutions in healthcare in EU, US, China, and Russia: new scenarios after a pandemic. *Radiation*, 1, 261–276.

40. Pesapane F, Volonté C, Codari M, Sardanelli F. (2018) Artificial intelligence as a medical device in radiology: ethical and regulatory issues in Europe and the United States. *Insights Imaging*, **9**, 745–753.

41. (2021) WHO issues first global report on Artificial Intelligence (AI) in health and six guiding principles for its design and use. https://www.who.int/news/item/28-06-2021-who-issues-first-global-report-on-ai-in-health-and-six-guiding-principles-for-its-design-and-use

42. IEEE standard model process for addressing ethical concerns during system design. https://standards.ieee.org/ieee/7000/6781/

43. (2022) The Belmont Report. https://www.hhs.gov/ohrp/regulations-and-policy/belmont-report/index.html

44. Morley J, Machado CCV, Burr C, Cowls J, Joshi I, Taddeo M, Floridi L. (2020) The ethics of AI in health care: a mapping review. *Social Science & Medicine*, **260**, 113172.

45. Bruce G. (2023) 41.4 million affected by healthcare data breaches this year, nearing '22 totals. https://www.beckershospitalreview.com/cybersecurity/41-4-million-affected-by-healthcare-data-breaches-this-year-nearing-22-to-tals.html#:~:text=Healthcare%20organizations%20have%20reported%20330,affected%20nearly%2016%20million%20patients

46. Alder S. (2022) Study reveals one third of top 100 U.S. hospitals are sending patient data to Facebook. https://www.hipaajournal.com/study-reveals-one-third-of-top-100-u-s-hospitals-are-sending-patient-data-to-facebook/#:~:text=Data%20to%20Facebook-,Study%20Reveals%20One%20Third%20of%20Top%20100%20U.S.,Sending%20Patient%20Data%20to%20Facebook&text=An%20analysis%20of%20hospitals'%20websites,apparently%20obtaining%20consent%20from%20patients

47. Ledford H. (2019) Millions of black people affected by racial bias in healthcare algorithms. *Nature*, **574**(7780), 608–609.

48. Topol EJ. (2019) High-performance medicine: the convergence of human and artificial intelligence. *Nature Medicine*, **25**, 44–56.

Chapter 9

Regulatory and Legal Frameworks for AI in Medicine

Introduction

On May 16th, 2023, in a hearing of the Senate Judiciary Committee on the topic of artificial intelligence (AI), Sam Altman, CEO of OpenAI, said that there was a need for "a new agency that licenses any effort above a certain scale of capabilities and could take that license away and ensure compliance with safety standards."[1] When a leader of any industry pleads with the government for more regulation, it suggests that there might be a cause for concern. Mr. Altman's request emphasizes the dangers associated with this new technology and the need for safety standards.

Therefore, as the field of medicine embraces the transformative potential of AI, it is essential to establish robust regulatory and legal frameworks to guide its implementation.[2] For healthcare professionals, navigating the complex landscape of AI regulations and guidelines can be challenging. This chapter aims to provide an overview of existing regulations and guidelines governing the use of AI in healthcare and address the specific concerns relevant to clinicians. We will delve into the challenges of developing regulatory frameworks for AI, including privacy, security, liability, and intellectual property issues. By understanding the regulatory compliance and guidelines for AI development and deployment, as well as the implications of privacy and data security in AI applications, healthcare professionals can confidently embrace the benefits of AI in medicine while ensuring patient safety and ethical practice.

Overview of existing regulations and guidelines governing the use of AI in healthcare

To promote responsible and ethical use of AI in medicine, comprehensive regulations and clear guidelines should be established. Here we will explore key regulations and guidelines, providing real-world examples that highlight the importance of these measures in safeguarding patient well-being and maintaining trust in AI-driven healthcare.

Regulatory bodies and guidelines

Numerous regulatory bodies and organizations have issued guidelines to address the ethical and legal challenges associated with AI in healthcare.[3,4] The U.S. government is still in the early stages of developing a comprehensive regulatory framework for AI. However, there have been a number of recent developments that signal a growing interest in regulating AI (e.g., Executive Order on the Safe, Secure, and Trustworthy Development and Use of Artificial Intelligence). In October 2023, President Biden signed an executive order on AI that outlines five principles for the development and use of AI:

1. AI should be developed and deployed in a way that is safe and reliable.
2. AI should be accessible to everyone, regardless of background or identity.
3. AI should be used to promote fairness and equity.
4. AI should be respectful of privacy and civil liberties.
5. AI should be accountable to the people it serves.

The executive order also establishes an Artificial Intelligence Risk Management Framework to help agencies assess and mitigate the risks of AI systems. Additionally, it creates an Artificial Intelligence Safety and Security Board to advise the Department of Homeland Security on AI safety and security issues. The U.S. national approach to AI regulation, so far, involves delegating responsibilities to specific federal agencies. While comprehensive regulation of AI is not pursued, federal agencies, such as the United States Food and Drug Administration (FDA), play a leadership role in formulating regulatory guidance for AI applications in medicine. The FDA has been actively involved in regulating AI in medical products. They have defined AI as "the science and engineering of making intelligent machines" and have issued guidelines to ensure the safety and effectiveness of AI-enabled healthcare products.[5] Another example is the Ministry of Health (MOH) in Singapore. The MOH, in collaboration with the Health Sciences Authority (HSA) and the Integrated Health Information Systems (IHiS), has developed the MOH Artificial Intelligence in Healthcare Guidelines (AIHGle).[6] These guidelines aim to promote the safe design and implementation of AI in healthcare, emphasizing good practices for both AI developers and implementers.

Ethical challenges and informed consent

One of the primary ethical challenges in AI-driven healthcare is obtaining informed consent from patients.[7] The use of AI algorithms may involve the processing of sensitive patient data, raising concerns about privacy and data protection. Regulations, such as the European Union's General Data Protection Regulation (GDPR), provide a framework for protecting patient data and ensuring informed consent for AI applications.[8,9] Implemented on May 25th, 2018, the GDPR imposes obligations on organizations globally if they target or collect data of individuals in the EU. It sets privacy and security standards for handling personal data and includes provisions for significant fines, reaching into the tens of millions of euros, to penalize violations of these standards.

Algorithmic bias and transparency

To address the issue of algorithmic bias, regulations are being developed to ensure transparency and accountability in AI systems. The European Union (EU) has proposed the Artificial Intelligence Act (AIA) to promote transparency and explainability in AI algorithms, particularly in critical healthcare applications.[10] The AIA emphasizes the importance of addressing biases that may disproportionately impact certain patient groups. For practicing clinicians, the AIA's focus on transparency and explainability in AI algorithms can have significant implications. Here are a few relevant examples:

- Patient diagnosis: AI algorithms are increasingly used to assist healthcare professionals in diagnosing medical conditions. Transparency and explainability requirements can help ensure that clinicians have a clear understanding of how the AI system arrives at its diagnostic recommendations. This enables healthcare professionals to make more informed decisions and provides an opportunity to detect and address potential biases in the AI algorithms.

- Treatment recommendations: AI systems can aid clinicians in suggesting treatment plans based on patient data. With transparency and explainability requirements, physicians can better understand the underlying factors and considerations considered by the AI system. This allows them to critically evaluate the treatment recommendations and ensure that they align with their clinical expertise and the individual needs of patients.

- Clinical trials and research: AI algorithms are used in the analysis of large datasets for clinical trials and medical research. Transparency requirements can help healthcare professionals understand the specific data inputs and features that influence the AI's outcomes. This fosters trust in the AI system and allows clinicians to validate the reliability and generalizability of the AI-driven insights obtained from clinical trials and research.

- Bias mitigation: The AIA's emphasis on addressing biases is particularly relevant for clinicians. AI systems trained on biased or unrepresentative datasets can produce skewed results, leading to unequal healthcare outcomes. Transparency and accountability provisions can help identify and mitigate such biases, ensuring fair and unbiased treatment for all patient groups.

By promoting transparency and explainability in AI algorithms, the AIA empowers clinicians to make more informed decisions, improves patient outcomes, and safeguards against potential biases in AI-driven healthcare applications.

Safety and effectiveness

Regulatory frameworks in healthcare focus on ensuring the safety and effectiveness of AI technologies. As an example, Health Canada, the department of government of Canada responsible for national health policy, plays a role in regulating health-related AI products to address safety concerns and potential risks associated with algorithmic decision-making.[11] This approach is crucial in protecting patients and promoting responsible innovation in the field.

Healthcare professionals are directly involved in the implementation and use of AI technologies in healthcare. Here are examples that highlight the relevance of safety and effectiveness regulations for clinicians:

- Clinical decision support systems: AI-powered clinical decision support systems provide physicians with evidence-based recommendations for diagnosis, treatment, and patient management. Regulatory frameworks ensure that these systems undergo rigorous evaluation to validate their safety and effectiveness. Healthcare professionals can rely on these regulated AI systems to make informed decisions, enhancing patient care.
- Medical imaging analysis: AI algorithms are increasingly used for analyzing medical images such as X-rays, MRIs, and CT scans. Regulatory frameworks ensure that AI image analysis systems meet safety and effectiveness standards before being deployed in clinical settings. Clinicians benefit from these regulations by having access to reliable AI tools that assist in accurate and timely diagnoses.
- Personalized medicine: AI algorithms enable the analysis of large datasets to identify patterns and predict patient responses to specific treatments. Regulatory frameworks ensure that AI-driven personalized medicine approaches are safe and effective. Healthcare professionals can leverage these regulated AI tools to tailor treatments based on individual patient characteristics, optimizing outcomes.
- Adverse event monitoring: AI systems can be used to monitor and analyze real-time data from electronic health records and other sources to detect adverse events and potential risks. Regulatory frameworks emphasize the need for robust monitoring and reporting

mechanisms, enabling physicians to identify and respond to safety concerns promptly.

• Quality improvement initiatives: AI technologies assist healthcare professionals in analyzing healthcare data to identify trends, measure performance, and implement quality improvement initiatives. Regulatory frameworks ensure that AI-driven quality improvement processes are reliable and effective, empowering physicians to make data-driven decisions that enhance patient outcomes.

By focusing on the safety and effectiveness of AI technologies, regulatory frameworks provide physicians with the assurance that AI tools meet specific standards, can be trusted in clinical practice, and prioritize patient well-being.[12] These regulations foster responsible integration of AI in healthcare, enabling clinicians to leverage AI technologies to augment their expertise and improve patient care.

Standards and best practices

International standards organizations, such as the International Organization for Standardization (ISO), play a crucial role in developing standards and best practices for AI in healthcare.[13,14] These standards aim to ensure interoperability, data security, and the ethical use of AI technologies in medical settings. Physicians benefit from these standards in several ways:

• Interoperability: Standards facilitate the seamless integration of AI technologies into existing healthcare systems, allowing physicians to exchange data and insights across different platforms and devices. For example, ISO/IEEE 11073 Health informatics standards enable the interoperability of medical devices and health information systems, ensuring that data collected by AI systems can be effectively shared and utilized by physicians.[15]

• Data security and privacy: Standards address the critical concerns of data security and patient privacy when using AI technologies. They provide guidelines for secure data storage, transmission, and access control, protecting sensitive patient information. Compliance with standards such as ISO/IEC 27001 Information Security Management System helps physicians ensure the confidentiality, integrity, and availability of healthcare data processed by AI systems.[16]

- Ethical use of AI: Standards outline ethical principles and guidelines for the development and deployment of AI in healthcare. They help physicians navigate complex ethical considerations, ensuring the responsible and accountable use of AI technologies. The World Health Organization (WHO) has issued guiding principles for AI in healthcare, emphasizing the importance of ethics, human rights, and transparency in AI design and deployment.[17]

- Quality assurance: Standards assist physicians in evaluating the quality and reliability of AI technologies.[18] They define criteria for performance assessment, validation, and testing of AI algorithms and systems. By adhering to recognized standards, physicians can ensure that the AI technologies they employ meet established quality benchmarks, leading to reliable and accurate outcomes. Unfortunately, a comprehensive framework to systematically assess quality across all stages of AI-based prediction model development, evaluation and implementation is still lacking. The absence of this framework may be the reason why relatively few models have been implemented to date.[19]

- Regulatory compliance: Standards provide a framework for regulatory compliance in the field of AI in healthcare. Regulatory bodies, such as the U.S. Food and Drug Administration (FDA), often refer to international standards when evaluating the safety and effectiveness of AI-based medical products. Compliance with relevant standards can help physicians navigate regulatory requirements and ensure the proper use of AI technologies.

By following international standards, physicians can confidently adopt and utilize AI technologies in healthcare settings. These standards promote interoperability, safeguard patient data, ensure ethical practices, maintain quality standards, and aid regulatory compliance, ultimately contributing to improved patient care and outcomes.

Challenges and considerations in developing regulatory frameworks for AI

The development of regulatory frameworks for AI in healthcare presents unique challenges and considerations. As healthcare professionals, it is important to understand these complexities, even without a background in law or regulatory frameworks. This overview will discuss key challenges and considerations in developing regulatory frameworks for AI in healthcare, providing real-world examples to illustrate their significance.

Ethical and human rights implications

AI in healthcare raises ethical and human rights concerns, as highlighted by WHO.[17] Designing regulatory frameworks that prioritize ethics and human rights is crucial to ensure responsible AI deployment. For example, regulations should address issues like algorithmic bias, privacy protection, and the potential for AI to exacerbate existing healthcare disparities.

Balancing innovation and patient safety

Regulatory frameworks must strike a balance between promoting innovation and ensuring patient safety. AI technologies can greatly enhance healthcare delivery, but they also introduce new risks. Establishing clear guidelines for risk assessment, validation, and monitoring of AI systems is essential. The State of Regulation of Medical Software and AI report[20] emphasizes the need for a system that verifies the quality and safety of AI technologies.

Fairness and transparency

Developing regulatory frameworks that promote fairness and transparency is critical. Algorithms used in AI systems can be complex, making it challenging to understand how they arrive at decisions. Ensuring transparency in algorithmic decision-making is essential to building trust and addressing concerns about biased outcomes.

Collaboration and interoperability

Regulatory frameworks should foster collaboration and interoperability among stakeholders. AI applications often rely on interoperable data exchange and integration with existing healthcare systems.[21] However, most of the medical data available today suffers from a lack of interoperability: the data is siloed in isolated databases, incompatible systems, and proprietary software, making it challenging to exchange, analyze, and interpret. Coordinated efforts among regulatory bodies, healthcare providers, and technology developers are necessary to establish standards and protocols that enable seamless integration and data sharing. International organizations, such as the Organization for Economic Co-operation and Development (OECD), work toward aligning views on ethical and trustworthy AI to enhance cross-border interoperability.[22]

Adapting to rapid technological advancements

Regulatory frameworks for AI in healthcare must be flexible and adaptive to keep pace with rapidly evolving technologies. Traditional regulatory processes, built on assumptions more appropriate to the industrial era, may struggle to keep up with the fast-paced innovation in AI. Implementing mechanisms for continuous monitoring, evaluation, and iterative improvement of regulatory frameworks is imperative. The increasing challenges of regulating AI in healthcare is prompting regulators to reimagine the regulation rule book and nurture innovation.

Addressing privacy, security, and liability concerns related to AI adoption in medicine

The adoption of AI in medicine has the potential to revolutionize healthcare delivery but it also raises important concerns related to privacy, security, and liability. This following segment will address the key privacy, security, and liability concerns associated with AI adoption in medicine, providing real-world examples and clear arguments to elucidate their significance.

Privacy concerns

The first set of concerns revolves around access, use, and control of patient data in the hands of private entities. When AI technologies are owned and controlled by private corporations, hospitals, or clinics, the handling and protection of patient health information become critical privacy considerations. For instance, unauthorized access or breaches of patient data could lead to compromising sensitive medical information and violating patient privacy.

The rapid proliferation and integration of AI systems in healthcare has led to greater attention on privacy risks and safeguards. This heightened focus can be attributed to the swift expansion of healthcare AI, as well as collaborative efforts like the Health AI Partnership formed by organizations including DLA Piper, Mayo Clinic, and the Duke Institute for Health Innovations to address these concerns.[23] These initiatives aimed to establish guidelines and standards for responsible AI. Additionally, entities using AI-based healthcare products need to consider federal and state laws and regulations governing the collection and use of patient data to ensure compliance with privacy requirements, such as the Health Insurance Portability and Accountability Act (HIPAA).

Security concerns

AI adoption in medicine introduces new security challenges. The exchange of medical information between patients, physicians, and care teams through AI systems requires robust measures to protect the underlying data. Data breaches, cyber-attacks, and unauthorized access to AI systems pose significant risks, potentially compromising patient confidentiality and the integrity of healthcare processes.[24] From January 2016 to December 2021, 374 ransomware attacks on US health care delivery organizations exposed the personal health information of nearly 42 million patients.[25] Ransomware attacks against healthcare organizations doubled in the last five years, with the most common victim being health clinics, according to a JAMA Health Forum study.[26] When compared to other data industries such as banking, insurance, or social media companies, the healthcare industry is among the most effected by data breaches.[27] Ensuring the security of AI systems and safeguarding patient data are essential for maintaining trust and protecting sensitive medical information.

Liability concerns

The adoption of AI in medicine presents the possibility that algorithm-based errors could cause injury to patients. This raises liability concerns regarding accountability and responsibility for AI-driven decisions and actions. AI systems are designed to make autonomous decisions based on complex algorithms, which can create challenges when assigning liability for adverse outcomes. Determining who is responsible for AI errors, malfunctions, or misdiagnoses becomes crucial in maintaining patient safety and ensuring appropriate legal recourse.[28]

On one hand, it seems logical for developers to assume the risk of liability since they are the ones creating and implementing AI with the intention of improving medical care. If AI fails to perform as expected, patients are the ones who suffer, and accountability should be assigned to those responsible for the flawed product. This perspective suggests that developers should bear the liability for any harm caused by their AI systems. On the other hand, courts have been hesitant to extend product liability to software developers for several reasons. Firstly, AI is designed to assist healthcare providers in making informed decisions, not to replace their expertise. In the context of employing an AI system to make a diagnosis, the healthcare providers assume the role of the "learned intermediary."[29]

The learned intermediary doctrine is a legal principle that typically applies in cases involving prescription medical products, where the manufacturer has a duty to warn the prescribing healthcare professional (the learned intermediary) about the risks associated with the product. The healthcare professional then has the responsibility to convey those warnings to the patient. In the context of AI and medical diagnostics, the learned intermediary doctrine may be invoked to determine liability. If an AI system is used to assist in diagnosing a patient, the responsibility for conveying accurate information and warnings about the AI system's limitations would likely fall on the healthcare professional. The healthcare professional would be expected to exercise their own judgment, consider the AI system's recommendations alongside their own expertise, and communicate the diagnosis and associated risks to the patient.

If an erroneous diagnosis occurs due to a flaw or limitation in the AI system, the liability analysis would likely focus on whether the healthcare professional adequately considered and communicated the AI system's limitations to the patient. If it is determined that the healthcare professional failed to fulfill their duty to warn the patient or did not exercise proper judgment in relying on the AI system, they may bear some liability for the harm caused. Therefore, it is imperative for healthcare professionals to exercise discretion and be aware of potential flaws when using AI for diagnosis and treatment. If there is a risk of false diagnosis or treatment complications, the healthcare provider who relies solely on AI without confirming through their own knowledge and expertise should be held liable.

Another consideration of the courts would be "What would be the effect of high liability costs on the development of new AI systems?" Imposing liability on developers for any discrepancy could discourage the development of new modifications that could further enhance AI in healthcare. The fear of legal repercussions may hinder the growth of AI, which is why courts should exercise caution when determining developer liability. The promotion of new innovations in AI is essential for improving the healthcare industry. Fear of litigation should not impede this progress.

Therefore, clarifying liability frameworks and guidelines is necessary to establish accountability and ensure patient protection. Liability frameworks can be designed to strike a balance between encouraging innovation and safeguarding patient well-being. As an example, developers could be held liable if they fail to meet a reasonable standard of care in the development and deployment of their AI systems. This approach does not mean punishing developers for every minor discrepancy, but rather establishing a threshold that ensures due diligence and accountability. By addressing liability concerns, healthcare professionals can navigate potential legal challenges, allocate responsibilities, and establish clear standards for AI system development and use. Moreover, addressing liability issues promotes trust and confidence in AI technologies, which is vital for their widespread adoption in healthcare settings.

Intellectual property issues associated with the adoption of AI in medicine

What are intellectual property rights?

Intellectual property rights refer to the legal rights and protections granted to individuals or entities over their intangible creations of the mind.[30] These rights enable creators to have exclusive control over the use, distribution, and commercial exploitation of their intellectual creations, thereby providing an incentive for innovation, creativity, and investment. Intellectual property encompasses a wide range of intangible assets, including inventions, literary and artistic works, designs, symbols, names, images, trade secrets, trademarks, and patents.

The purpose of intellectual property rights is to strike a balance between the interests of innovators, creators, and the broader public. By granting exclusive rights to creators, intellectual property laws encourage the development and dissemination of new ideas, technologies, and creative works. At the same time, these laws aim to foster an environment where the public can benefit from the knowledge and cultural advancements derived from these creations.

Why are intellectual property rights important in AI?

In the context of AI adoption in medicine, intellectual property rights are critical because they provide legal protection for innovative AI technologies and inventions. Intellectual property rights, such as patents and copyrights, enable inventors and developers to safeguard their AI-related innovations, algorithms, and models. By protecting their intellectual property, healthcare organizations, and researchers can maintain a competitive advantage, encourage investment in AI research and development, and foster a culture of innovation within the medical field. Intellectual property rights also incentivize collaboration and knowledge-sharing while ensuring that AI technologies are used responsibly and ethically.

Intellectual property issues in AI adoption

The increasing use of AI in healthcare has raised important questions about copyright infringement and ownership of AI-generated content. As generative AI becomes prevalent in various industries, including healthcare, it is crucial to understand the challenges in determining copyright ownership and the legal implications of using generative AI and unlicensed content in training data.

Challenges in determining copyright ownership

Determining copyright ownership of AI-generated content poses significant challenges in healthcare. AI systems, such as generative AI platforms, utilize enormous datasets to discover patterns and relationships. The output generated by these systems can range from marketing materials for a new drug to content in a medical text. However, establishing who owns the copyright of such works becomes complex due to the involvement of AI algorithms in the creative process. Courts are currently grappling with the application of intellectual property laws to generative AI, and cases related to copyright infringement and ownership have already emerged.[31]

Legal implications of using generative AI and unlicensed content

The use of generative AI in healthcare raises legal implications, particularly concerning unlicensed content used in training data. Generative AI platforms rely on existing works to train their models and generate new content in response to prompts. However, incorporating copyrighted material without proper licenses in the training data can potentially lead to copyright infringement issues. The Copyright Act considers the reproduction or communication of a "substantial part" of a work as infringement, regardless of whether it was generated by AI or a human. Determining what constitutes a substantial part can be complex, especially in artistic works. Therefore, healthcare professionals must be cautious when using generative AI platforms and ensure compliance with copyright laws.

Navigating the legal landscape

Clinicians engaging with generative AI platforms and AI-generated content need to navigate the legal landscape surrounding copyright ownership and infringement. Understanding the source and legality of the content used in AI training data is essential to avoid copyright violations. Companies that provide generative AI platforms should have proper licensing agreements and ensure that their systems do not generate content that infringes on copyright. Healthcare professionals must be aware of the copyright implications and exercise due diligence when using AI-generated works in their practice.

Mitigating risks and ensuring compliance

To mitigate copyright risks and ensure compliance, healthcare organizations, and clinicians should consider the following measures:

- Implementing robust data governance: Healthcare organizations should establish stringent data governance protocols to ensure that AI training data does not include unlicensed copyrighted materials.
- Seeking proper licensing: When using generative AI platforms, clinicians should verify that the platforms have obtained appropriate licenses for the training data, ensuring that copyrighted works are used with permission.
- Monitoring AI-generated content: Clinicians should regularly monitor the output of generative AI systems to identify and address any potential copyright infringement issues. Implementing content filtering mechanisms can help identify unlicensed content.
- Engaging legal expertise: Healthcare organizations and physicians should consult legal experts specializing in intellectual property law to navigate the complexities of copyright ownership and infringement in the context of AI-generated content.

By understanding and complying with copyright laws, practicing healthcare professionals can harness the benefits of generative AI while respecting intellectual property rights and legal obligations.

Conclusion

The adoption of AI in medicine requires a comprehensive approach to address intellectual property and liability issues. Developing frameworks and guidelines that prioritize ethics, human rights, and responsible use of AI in healthcare is crucial. By navigating these challenges effectively, we can unlock the transformative potential of AI while ensuring patient safety, privacy, and equitable access to healthcare. It is through collaborative efforts and the integration of multidisciplinary expertise that we can shape a future where AI in medicine benefits society.

References

1. Tracy R. (2023) ChatGPT's Sam Altman warns congress that AI 'can go quite wrong'. https://www.wsj.com/articles/chatgpts-sam-altman-faces-senate-panel-examining-artificial-intelligence-4bb6942a
2. Khan B, Fatima H, Qureshi A, Kumar S, Hanan A, Hussain J, Abdullah S. (2023) Drawbacks of artificial intelligence and their potential solutions in the healthcare sector. Biomed Mater Devices, 8, 1–8.
3. Naik N, Hameed BMZ, Shetty DK, Swain D, Shah M, Paul R, Aggarwal K, Ibrahim S, Patil V, Smriti K, Shetty S, Rai BP, Chlosta P, Somani BK. (2022) Legal and ethical consideration in artificial intelligence in healthcare: who takes responsibility? *Frontiers in Surgery*, **9**, 862322.
4. (2021) How FDA regulates artificial intelligence in medical products. https://www.pewtrusts.org/en/research-and-analysis/issue-briefs/2021/08/how-fda-regulates-artificial-intelligence-in-medical-products
5. (2021) Artificial intelligence and machine learning in software as a medical device. https://www.fda.gov/medical-devices/software-medical-device-samd/artificial-intelligence-and-machine-learning-software-medical-device
6. Artificial intelligence in healthcare. https://www.moh.gov.sg/licensing-and-regulation/artificial-intelligence-in-healthcare
7. Farhud DD, Zokaei S. (2021) Ethical issues of artificial intelligence in medicine and healthcare. *Iranian Journal of Public Health*, **50**(11), i–v.

8. Meszaros J, Minari J, Huys I. (2022) The future regulation of artificial intelligence systems in healthcare services and medical research in the European Union. Frontiers in Genetics, **13**, 927721.

9. Lekadir K, *et al.* (2022) Artificial intelligence in healthcare: applications, risks, and ethical and societal impacts. https://www.europarl.europa.eu/RegData/etudes/STUD/2022/729512/EPRS_STU(2022)729512_EN.pdf

10. van Oirschot J, Ooms G. (2022) Interpreting the EU Artificial Intelligence Act for the health sector. https://haiweb.org/wp-content/uploads/2022/02/Interpreting-the-EU-Artificial-Intelligence-Act-for-the-Health-Sector.pdf

11. Da Silva M, Flood CM, Goldenberg A, Singh D. (2022) Regulating the safety of health-related artificial intelligence. *Healthcare policy = Politiques de sante*, **17**(4), 63–77.

12. He J, Baxter SL, Xu J, Xu J, Zhou X, Zhang K. (2019) The practical implementation of artificial intelligence technologies in medicine. *Nature Medicine*, **25**(1), 30–36.

13. Kerry CF, *et al.* (2021) Strengthening international cooperation on AI. https://www.brookings.edu/articles/strengthening-international-cooperation-on-ai/

14. Glickman M. (2023) How AI drives innovation in healthcare. https://www.iso.org/contents/news/2023/04/ai-in-healthcare.html

15. Health informatics — Device interoperability — Part 20701: Point-of-care medical device communication — Service oriented medical device exchange architecture and protocol binding. https://www.iso.org/obp/ui/en/#iso:std:iso-ieee:11073:-20701:ed-1:v1:en

16. ISO 27701: The international standard for privacy information management. https://www.itgovernanceusa.com/iso-27701

17. (2021) WHO issues first global report on Artificial Intelligence (AI) in health and six guiding principles for its design and use. https://www.who.int/news/item/28-06-2021-who-issues-first-global-report-on-ai-in-health-and-six-guiding-principles-for-its-design-and-use accessed 8/15/23

18. de Hond AAH, Leeuwenberg AM, Hooft L, *et al.* (2022) Guidelines and quality criteria for artificial intelligence-based prediction models in healthcare: a scoping review. *npj Digital Medicine*, **5**, 2.

19. Collins GS, Reitsma JB, Altman DG, Moons KGM. (2015) Transparent reporting of a multivariable prediction model for individual prognosis or diagnosis (TRIPOD): The TRIPOD Statement. *European Urology*, **67**, 1142–1151.

20. Brown N, Kessler C. The state of regulation of medical software and AI: considerations for clinicians and providers. https://sharepoint.healthlawyers.org/find-a-resource/HealthLawHub/Documents/AI/III_Regulation_The%20

State%20of%20Regulation%20of%20Medical%20Software%20and%20
AI%20Considerations%20for%20Clinicians%20and%20Providers.pdf

21. Lehne M, Sass J, Essenwanger A, *et al.* (2019) Why digital medicine depends on interoperability. *npj Digital Medicine*, **2**, 79.

22. Artificial intelligence. https://www.oecd.org/digital/artificial-intelligence/

23. Kagan D, *et al.* (2023) Industry organizations establish practical frameworks for digital health and healthcare AI tools. https://www.lexology.com/library/detail.aspx?g=e0ed64f4-da94-4343-a732-09e4cccb8f2b

24. Seh AH, Zarour M, Alenezi M, Sarkar AK, Agrawal A, Kumar R, Khan RA. (2020) Healthcare data breaches: insights and implications. *Healthcare (Basel)*, **8**(2), 133.

25. Neprash HT, McGlave CC, Cross DA, Virnig BA, Puskarich MA, Huling JD, Rozenshtein AZ, Nikpay SS. (2022) Trends in ransomware attacks on us hospitals, clinics, and other health care delivery organizations, 2016-2021. *JAMA Health Forum*, **3**(12), e224873.

26. Burky A. (2023) Researchers crawled search engines and searched the dark web to find out the true extent of healthcare ransomware attacks. https://www.fiercehealthcare.com/health-tech/new-jama-study-scrapes-dark-web-find-true-frequency-healthcare-ransomware-attacks

27. Liu V, Musen MA, Chou T. (2015) Data breaches of protected health information in the United States. *JAMA Network*, **313**, 1471–1473.

28. Gerke S, Minssen T, Cohen G. (2020) Ethical and legal challenges of artificial intelligence-driven healthcare. *Artificial Intelligence in Healthcare*, **2020**, 295–336.

29. Price WN 2nd, Gerke S, Cohen IG. (2019) Potential liability for physicians using artificial intelligence. *JAMA Network*, **322**(18), 1765 –1766.

30. What are intellectual property rights? https://www.wto.org/english/tratop_e/trips_e/intel1_e.htm

31. United States Copyright Office. (2023) Copyright Registration Guidance: works containing material generated by artificial intelligence. https://www.copyright.gov/ai/ai_policy_guidance.pdf

Chapter 10

Healthcare Worker Displacement in the Era of AI

"I think that if you work as a radiologist, you are like Wile E. Coyote in the cartoon. You're already over the edge of the cliff, but you haven't yet looked down. There's no ground underneath. It's just completely obvious that in five years deep learning is going to do better than radiologists. It might be ten years."

Geoffrey Hinton, Cognitive Scientist and Pioneering Computer Scientist

Introduction

In recent years, the adoption of artificial intelligence (AI) technologies in healthcare has gained significant momentum. AI has the potential to transform the practice of medicine, improve patient outcomes, and enhance the delivery of healthcare services. However, alongside these advancements, there is growing concern about the potential displacement of workers due to the integration of AI systems.[1,2] Indeed, a 2023 report from Goldman Sachs estimated that around 300 million jobs worldwide could be automated by generative AI.[3] Advanced economies are predicted to be more heavily impacted than emerging markets. In the same report, analysts at Goldman Sachs predicted that more than 28% of U.S. healthcare practitioners are at risk to be displaced by AI systems. The objective of this chapter is to examine the factors contributing to healthcare worker displacement caused by the adoption of AI and propose strategies to mitigate its effects.

Job displacement refers to the situation in which AI systems, through automation and technological advancements, take over tasks and roles traditionally performed by human workers, leading to a reduced need for human involvement in those specific tasks.[4] This phenomenon is a result of the ongoing development and implementation of AI technologies across various industries. One of the significant drivers of job displacement is the increasing capability of AI systems to perform tasks that were previously exclusive to human workers. AI technologies, such as machine learning algorithms and robotics, have demonstrated the ability to perform tasks more efficiently, accurately, and tirelessly compared to humans in certain contexts. This can lead to the restructuring of industries and organizations as they adopt AI-powered solutions to streamline operations and cut costs.

The rapid progress in AI technology, particularly in areas such as medical diagnosis, personalized treatment plans, and administrative tasks, has led to the automation of certain healthcare tasks that were traditionally performed by human professionals. For instance, AI systems are being used to analyze medical imaging scans, assisting radiologists in diagnosing diseases. As Maryann Hardy says in her 2020 British Journal of Radiology article,[5] "Considering the current range of tasks that radiographers perform within cross-sectional imaging, and cross-mapping these with proposed areas for AI automation, it is clear that AI is poised to assist the radiographers' role significantly. However, such a level of automation, if achieved in full, could also significantly reduce current radiographer roles and responsibilities." Similarly, AI-powered chatbots are being employed to schedule appointments, answer questions about insurance coverage, triage patient inquiries and provide initial medical advice, reducing the need for human intervention in certain cases.[6,7] These examples demonstrate the transformative potential of AI in healthcare while raising questions about the future role of healthcare professionals.

By exploring the potential for healthcare worker displacement caused by AI adoption, we can better understand the challenges and opportunities associated with this technological revolution. This chapter aims to contribute to the ongoing discussions on AI in healthcare by shedding light on the implications for the healthcare workforce and proposing strategies to mitigate displacement effects. Ultimately, it is important to strike a balance between leveraging the benefits of AI and ensuring the continued involvement and reimagining of healthcare professionals in the delivery of patient-centered care.

Understanding the dynamics of healthcare worker displacement

With the expanding adoption of AI, its impact on the healthcare workforce is becoming more significant. The integration of AI systems in healthcare can result in job displacement, where AI fully replaces human workers, as well as job transformation, where tasks are redistributed between humans and AI. In the context of physicians, healthcare worker displacement due to AI implementation could involve AI systems taking over certain diagnostic or administrative tasks traditionally performed by physicians, thereby changing their roles and responsibilities. As AI reduces the amount of clinical tasks from physicians, fewer physicians are needed to perform the remaining tasks.

One example of healthcare worker displacement involving physicians is the use of AI-powered diagnostic systems. AI algorithms are involved in analyzing medical images, such as X-rays and MRIs, to detect abnormalities or assist in diagnosing diseases.[8] By leveraging AI for image analysis, physicians may experience a transformation in their role as they collaborate with AI systems to interpret and validate the results provided by the algorithms. Rather than solely relying on their own visual analysis, physicians can benefit from the ability of AI to quickly analyze vast amounts of medical images and provide potential diagnoses, enabling more efficient and accurate decision-making in patient care. With advances in clinical decision support AI models, healthcare organizations may choose to assign physician roles to a lower-paid medical professional, such as a nurse practitioner or physician assistant, with guidance provided by AI.[9,10] The feasibility of this decision hinges on whether doctors' responsibilities can be distilled into standardized questions and responses, or if they necessitate a greater level of expertise and nuanced decision-making.

These examples illustrate how the implementation of AI in healthcare can transform the tasks and responsibilities of physicians while still leveraging their expertise in conjunction with AI capabilities.

Estimating the size of healthcare worker displacement

Estimating how many healthcare workers could be displaced is a challenging and multifaceted task. It requires examining various aspects, including analyzing the workforce, assessing how jobs are changing, conducting cost-benefit analyses, and evaluating performance and productivity.[11] These evaluations are not only expensive but also complex, and there are few organizations with the motivation or resources to carry them out.

Factors contributing to displacement

Several factors contribute to healthcare worker displacement caused by AI implementation. Automation plays a significant role by automating repetitive and routine tasks that were previously performed by healthcare professionals. For example, AI algorithms can analyze medical imaging scans, such as X-rays and CT scans, to assist radiologists in diagnosing diseases. Machine learning algorithms enable AI systems to learn from clinical data and make predictions or recommendations, potentially replacing certain diagnostic or treatment decision-making processes traditionally performed by healthcare professionals. Robotics also play a role in displacement, with the introduction of robotic surgical systems that can perform precise surgical procedures under the guidance of human surgeons.

Traditional surgeries depend on the surgeon's eye to gather information about a lesion. However, human visualization has limitations. Image guidance technologies (e.g., computer vision) utilize AI image processing to analyze lesions and guide surgeons during procedures, overcoming the constraints of human vision alone.[12] The use of technologies like computer vision in surgery can shorten the duration of surgical cases and improve outcomes. The shorter the operative time, the fewer the number of surgeons needed to handle the workload.

Scope and scale of displacement across healthcare professions

The potential scope and scale of displacement vary across healthcare professions. Certain tasks within professions such as radiology, pathology, and dermatology can be automated or assisted by AI algorithms, leading to a shift in the role of healthcare professionals in these fields. For instance, the implementation of AI systems in radiology can facilitate the analysis of medical images, leading to a reduced workload for radiologists. AI algorithms can efficiently process and interpret medical images, allowing radiologists to focus on more complex or critical cases. By saving time and effort for radiologists, AI systems enable individual radiologists to read larger numbers of images within a given timeframe.

However, it is important to acknowledge that while one radiologist may benefit from AI assistance and the ability to read more images, other radiologists may experience underemployment or unemployment due to the reduced workload. The introduction of AI in radiology creates a shift in the distribution of work among radiologists, thereby warranting consideration of the broader implications for the radiology workforce, as was noted by Dr. Hinton in the quote at the beginning of this chapter.

Similarly, AI-powered chatbots can triage patient inquiries and provide initial medical advice, potentially reducing the workload of primary care physicians. Yet, it is important to note that AI systems are currently limited in their ability to replace complex decision-making, empathy, and the human touch required in patient care.

Distinction between job displacement and job transformation

A vital distinction exists between job displacement and job transformation in the context of healthcare worker AI displacement. Job displacement occurs when AI systems completely replace human workers, eliminating the need for their involvement in specific tasks. This can be seen in examples where AI algorithms directly analyze medical images or provide diagnoses without human intervention. In contrast, job transformation involves the redistribution of tasks between humans and AI. In this scenario, healthcare professionals collaborate with AI systems to enhance their capabilities and augment their decision-making processes. As an example, AI algorithms can assist physicians in diagnosing and treating diseases by providing additional insights or treatment recommendations, leading to a transformed role for healthcare professionals.

Comparing healthcare worker displacement with other industries affected by AI

The displacement of workers by AI is not unique to the healthcare industry. Various sectors including manufacturing, customer service, warehouse operations, and transportation have witnessed the displacement of human workers as AI and automation technologies advanced. For example, in manufacturing, robots have taken over repetitive assembly line tasks previously performed by human workers, leading to job displacement.[13] Similarly, automated customer service systems and chatbots have replaced human customer service representatives in certain industries, transforming the nature of customer interactions.[14]

Real-world examples of healthcare workers displaced by AI systems

Numerous real-world examples demonstrate the displacement of healthcare workers by AI systems. In addition to radiology mentioned above, pathology is another field where AI is making strides, with algorithms capable of analyzing histopathology slides and identifying cancerous cells or tumor markers.[15] Additionally, AI-powered virtual assistants and chatbots are being utilized in primary care settings to handle basic patient inquiries and triage, reducing the workload on physicians, and potentially leading to job transformation.[16]

Healthcare worker displacement is a significant concern in the era of AI implementation. Automation, machine learning algorithms, and robotics contribute to displacement by automating routine tasks, supporting decision-making, and performing surgical procedures. The scope and scale of displacement vary across healthcare professions, with some tasks being automated or transformed through collaboration with AI systems. The distinction between job displacement and job transformation is crucial in understanding the dynamics of healthcare worker displacement. While AI presents opportunities for improved efficiency and patient outcomes, it is important to strike a balance that preserves the human touch and ensures the reimagining of healthcare professionals' roles. Comparisons can be drawn between healthcare worker displacement and worker displacement in other industries affected by AI, highlighting common challenges and potential mitigation strategies. By examining real-world examples, we can better comprehend the dynamics of healthcare worker displacement and work towards strategies that promote the successful integration of AI in healthcare while preserving the value and expertise of healthcare professionals.

Assessing the impact of AI on healthcare roles and tasks

In this section, we will explore the impact of AI on healthcare workforce management, focusing on specific healthcare roles and tasks susceptible to displacement. We will also provide examples of AI applications that are already replacing or augmenting certain healthcare tasks. Additionally, we will discuss the potential benefits and challenges associated with the use of AI in healthcare workforce management, considering different healthcare professions such as nurses, radiologists, and administrative staff.

Susceptible healthcare roles and displacement by AI

AI technologies have the potential to automate and streamline various healthcare tasks, leading to the displacement or redistribution of certain roles among healthcare professionals. Administrative tasks, such as data entry, report writing, and appointment scheduling, can be efficiently handled by AI-powered systems, reducing the burden on administrative staff. This is in addition to tasks related to image interpretation in radiology and pathology.

In nursing, AI-powered virtual assistants can provide patient monitoring, personalized care plans, and reminders for medication adherence, enhancing patient experience and outcomes.[17] AI is also utilized in drug discovery, clinical decision support systems, and predictive analytics, aiding physicians in treatment planning and disease management.

Benefits of AI adoption in healthcare workforce management

The adoption of AI in healthcare workforce management offers several potential benefits. Firstly, AI technologies can improve efficiency by automating repetitive and time-consuming tasks, allowing healthcare professionals to focus on more complex and critical aspects of patient care. AI-powered systems can enhance accuracy in diagnosis and treatment planning, reducing errors and improving patient outcomes. Furthermore, AI can contribute to workforce optimization by redistributing tasks and improving resource allocation, leading to better workload management and patient care coordination.

Challenges of AI adoption in healthcare workforce management

While the benefits of AI in healthcare are substantial, challenges and limitations must be addressed. Data privacy and security concerns arise with the use of AI, as patient information needs to be safeguarded against unauthorized access and breaches. Ethical considerations are vital to ensure transparency, fairness, and accountability in AI algorithms and decision-making processes. Workforce disruption due to AI adoption should be managed carefully to mitigate potential job displacement. Healthcare professionals may require appropriate training and upskilling to effectively utilize AI technologies and understand their limitations.

AI has the potential to significantly impact healthcare workforce management by automating tasks, improving accuracy, and optimizing resource allocation. While certain roles and tasks may be susceptible to displacement, the benefits of AI adoption, such as increased efficiency and improved patient outcomes, are substantial. It is crucial for healthcare organizations to carefully navigate the challenges associated with AI, including data privacy, ethics, and workforce transition, to fully leverage the potential of AI in healthcare workforce management. By embracing AI technologies while considering the unique requirements of different healthcare professions, healthcare organizations can enhance the overall delivery of care and improve patient outcomes.

Ethical and social implications of healthcare worker displacement

The displacement of healthcare workers raises ethical concerns related to job loss and its impact on individuals and communities. Job loss can lead to economic hardships, contributing to disparities in income and access to resources. This can result in social consequences such as increased poverty, reduced social mobility, and a decline in overall well-being. Moreover, job displacement can disrupt social networks and communities, causing a loss of identity and a sense of belonging. Therefore, it is essential to address these ethical concerns to ensure a just and equitable society.

Impact on patient-provider relationships and quality of care

Healthcare worker displacement can have implications for patient-provider relationships and the quality of care. Continuity of care is critical for building trust and maintaining effective communication between patients and healthcare professionals. Displacement may disrupt these relationships, leading to reduced patient satisfaction and potentially compromising patient outcomes. Moreover, the loss of experienced healthcare workers can result in a decline in the quality of care, as expertise and institutional knowledge are essential for delivering effective and efficient healthcare services. Efforts must be made to preserve the patient-provider bond and ensure the provision of high-quality care during periods of displacement.

Responsibility of healthcare organizations and policymakers

Healthcare organizations and policymakers are responsible of mitigating the negative effects of healthcare worker displacement. Healthcare organizations should prioritize the well-being of their workforce and provide support mechanisms such as retraining programs, career transition assistance, and mental health support services. They should also promote workforce resilience and develop strategies to retain skilled healthcare professionals. Policymakers play a crucial role in implementing policies that address economic disparities and support job creation in the healthcare sector. They should also advocate for social safety nets, retraining opportunities, and policies that promote fair labor practices and reduce socioeconomic inequalities.

Social implications and consequences for workers and society

The displacement of healthcare workers can have far-reaching social implications. For healthcare workers, displacement can lead to feelings of insecurity, loss of professional identity, and increased stress and anxiety.[18] The psychological impact of displacement should be acknowledged and access to mental health support should be prioritized. Displacement can also widen socioeconomic disparities, as marginalized communities may bear a disproportionate burden of job loss and reduced access to healthcare services. Society at large may experience the consequences of a strained healthcare system, including decreased healthcare capacity and potential gaps in service delivery. Efforts to minimize these social implications should focus on retraining and upskilling opportunities, ensuring equitable access to healthcare, and promoting inclusive policies that address social inequalities.

Strategies for managing healthcare worker displacement

As AI technology continues to advance, strategies need to be developed to manage the potential displacement of healthcare workers.

Approaches for reskilling and upskilling healthcare workers

To successfully adapt to the AI-driven healthcare landscape, healthcare workers, particularly physicians, can benefit from reskilling and upskilling initiatives.[19] Training programs can be developed to equip them with the necessary skills to work alongside AI technologies. For example, physicians can be trained to interpret AI-generated insights, leverage AI algorithms for clinical decision-making, and understand the limitations and ethical considerations of AI in healthcare. Additionally, they can be trained in utilizing AI-powered tools and technologies for data analysis and interpretation. These reskilling and upskilling initiatives will ensure that healthcare workers remain relevant and valuable contributors to the healthcare system.

Importance of fostering a culture of continuous learning

Fostering a culture of continuous learning is vital in the AI-driven healthcare landscape. Clinicians will need to embrace continuous learning and regularly acquire new knowledge and skills throughout their careers as AI becomes integrated into healthcare.[20] This includes developing proficiency in utilizing, critically assessing, and enhancing AI systems. Building expertise in harnessing data analytics and intelligent technologies will be a crucial requirement for clinicians moving forward.

Healthcare organizations should provide opportunities for physicians to engage in ongoing professional development and stay updated with the latest advancements in AI and healthcare. This can be accomplished through workshops, conferences, online courses, and collaborative learning platforms.

By encouraging physicians to embrace lifelong learning, organizations can foster a dynamic workforce that adapts to technological advancements and maintains a high standard of care. Continuous learning also enables physicians to explore new roles and responsibilities within the healthcare system, enhancing their professional growth and job satisfaction.

Opportunities for transitioning and leveraging skills in the AI ecosystem

The integration of AI in healthcare presents opportunities for healthcare workers to transition into new roles and leverage their skills.[19] Physicians can explore positions as AI consultants, where they collaborate with AI developers and researchers to guide the development and implementation of AI solutions in healthcare. They can also become AI champions within their organizations, helping their peers understand and embrace the benefits of AI technology. Additionally, physicians can focus on patient-centered roles that require human empathy, clinical expertise, critical thinking, and complex decision-making, complementing the capabilities of AI algorithms. For instance, they can specialize in personalized care planning, end-of-life counseling, and ethical decision-making, where human judgment and emotional intelligence are essential. By leveraging their expertise and combining it with AI capabilities, physicians can play a crucial role in delivering high-quality, patient-centric care.

Additional strategies for managing displacement

In addition to reskilling and transitioning, other strategies can be employed to manage healthcare worker displacement. Job rotation programs can be implemented, allowing healthcare professionals to gain exposure to different areas of healthcare and develop new skills that align with the AI ecosystem. Redeployment initiatives can also be explored, where healthcare workers are assigned to different departments or specialties that are experiencing high demand. This enables them to contribute their expertise while adapting to changing healthcare needs. Furthermore, healthcare organizations can create new hybrid roles that blend human and AI capabilities. For example, physicians can work alongside AI-powered diagnostic tools, combining their clinical expertise with the efficiency and accuracy of AI algorithms.

The role of policymakers and healthcare organizations

Policymakers and healthcare organizations have a crucial role in managing healthcare worker displacement due to AI implementation. Policymakers should collaborate with industry experts and professional associations to develop supportive policies and regulations that address the ethical implications, privacy concerns, and workforce challenges associated with AI in healthcare. They can establish funding programs to support reskilling and upskilling initiatives, promote interdisciplinary research and innovation, and ensure a fair transition for displaced healthcare workers. Healthcare organizations should create supportive environments that encourage innovation, collaboration, and knowledge sharing. They can invest in AI infrastructure and technologies while simultaneously prioritizing the well-being and professional growth of their workforce. By aligning policies and organizational strategies, policymakers and healthcare organizations can facilitate a smooth transition to the AI-driven healthcare landscape.

Collaboration and partnerships in mitigating displacement effects

To effectively mitigate the effects of healthcare worker displacement, collaboration among stakeholders such as healthcare organizations, educational institutions, government agencies, professional associations, unions, and healthcare workers themselves is critical.

The need for collaboration among stakeholder

Collaboration among stakeholders is essential in addressing the challenges associated with displacement. Healthcare organizations, educational institutions, and government agencies should work together to develop comprehensive strategies and programs that support displaced healthcare workers in their career transitions. By sharing resources, expertise, and insights, stakeholders can collectively address the needs of displaced workers and ensure a smooth transition to new roles and responsibilities.

Strategies for fostering partnerships

To foster partnerships that support displaced healthcare workers, stakeholders can implement various strategies. Firstly, they can establish collaborative platforms where stakeholders can exchange ideas, best practices, and resources. These platforms can take the form of regular meetings, conferences, or online forums. Secondly, stakeholders can develop joint training programs that provide reskilling and upskilling opportunities for displaced workers. By pooling their resources, educational institutions and healthcare organizations can offer comprehensive training that aligns with the evolving needs of the healthcare industry. Lastly, stakeholders can establish mentorship programs that pair displaced healthcare workers with experienced professionals who can guide them through their career transitions.

Several successful initiatives and programs have been implemented to mitigate the effects of displacement. One example is the collaboration between healthcare organizations and educational institutions to develop accelerated training programs for displaced healthcare workers. These programs provide intensive training in emerging areas such as AI integration, data analysis, and telemedicine, equipping workers with the skills needed to thrive in the evolving healthcare landscape. Another example is the establishment of career transition centers, where healthcare workers receive personalized career coaching, job placement assistance, and access to educational resources. These centers serve as centralized hubs that facilitate collaboration among multiple stakeholders, including professional associations, unions, and educational institutions.

Role of professional associations, unions, and educational institutions

Professional associations, unions, and educational institutions play a crucial role in facilitating collaboration and supporting displaced healthcare workers. Professional associations can serve as advocates for displaced workers, ensuring their voices are heard in policy discussions and decision-making processes. They can also establish mentorship programs, networking events, and continuing education opportunities to support professional growth and career transitions. Unions can negotiate for benefits and resources that specifically address the needs of displaced workers, such as financial assistance for training or preferential job placement arrangements. Educational institutions can collaborate with healthcare organizations to develop tailored training programs and certifications that address the skill gaps faced by displaced workers.

Conclusion

This chapter highlights several key points. Firstly, it emphasizes the importance of proactive measures to address displacement and ensure a smooth transition for healthcare workers. As AI adoption in clinical medicine increases, stakeholders must anticipate and prepare for potential workforce changes. Secondly, the chapter advocates for ethical AI implementation, human-AI collaboration, and continuous support for the healthcare workforce. It emphasizes the need for AI to be designed and used in a manner that upholds ethics and human rights while leveraging the strengths of both humans and AI systems. Thirdly, the chapter suggests a comprehensive exploration of healthcare worker displacement, analyzing its challenges and implications, and proposing strategies to minimize negative effects and promote a sustainable and equitable AI-driven healthcare workforce. This holistic approach will contribute to a deeper understanding of the topic and provide actionable insights for stakeholders.

It is important to highlight the need for ongoing research, monitoring, and adaptation of strategies as AI continues to evolve in the healthcare industry. The rapid pace of technological advancements requires a dynamic approach to address healthcare worker displacement effectively. By conducting ongoing research, stakeholders can stay informed about the impact of AI on the workforce and make necessary adjustments to their strategies and policies. Additionally, the conclusion should underscore the significance of inclusivity and equity in AI implementation. Efforts should be made to ensure that the benefits of AI are accessible to all healthcare workers, regardless of their backgrounds or roles. By adopting a proactive and inclusive approach, the healthcare industry can navigate the challenges of displacement, harness the potential of AI, and build a sustainable future for healthcare workers and patients alike.

References

1. Davenport T, Kalakota R. (2019) The potential for artificial intelligence in healthcare. *Future Healthcare Journal*, **6**(2), 94–98.
2. AI and the health care workforce. https://www.aha.org/system/files/media/file/2019/09/Market_Insights_AI_Workforce_2.pdf
3. (2023) Generative AI could raise global GDP by 7%. https://www.goldmansachs.com/intelligence/pages/generative-ai-could-raise-global-gdp-by-7-percent.html
4. Autor DH. (2015) Why are there still so many jobs? The history and future of workplace automation. *Journal of Economic Perspectives*, **29**(3), 3–30.
5. Hardy M, Harvey H. (2020) Artificial intelligence in diagnostic imaging: impact on the radiography profession. *The British Journal of Radiology*, **93**(1108), 20190840.
6. Wilson L, Marasoiu M. (2022) The development and use of chatbots in public health: scoping review. *JMIR Human Factors*, **9**(4), e35882.
7. Benefits of chatbots in healthcare: 9 use cases of healthcare chatbots. https://www.inbenta.com/benefits-of-chatbots-in-healthcare-9-use-cases-of-healthcare-chatbots/
8. Tang X. (2019) The role of artificial intelligence in medical imaging research. *BJR Open*, **2**(1), 20190031.
9. Kwok R. (2023) Will AI eventually replace doctors? https://insight.kellogg.northwestern.edu/article/will-ai-replace-doctors
10. Tursunbayeva A, Renkema M. (2022) Artificial intelligence in health-care: implications for the job design of healthcare professionals. *Asia Pacific Journal of Human Resources*. https://doi.org/10.1111/1744-7941.12325
11. Marlar J. (2020) Assessing the impact of new technologies on the labor market: key constructs, gaps, and data collection strategies for the bureau of labor statistics. https://www.bls.gov/bls/congressional-reports/assessing-the-impact-of-new-technologies-on-the-labor-market.htm#3.3.0
12. Kitaguchi D, Takeshita N, Hasegawa H, Ito M. (2021) Artificial intelligence-based computer vision in surgery: recent advances and future perspectives. *Annals of Gastroenterological Surgery*, **6**(1), 29–36.
13. de Vries GJ, Gentile E, Miroudot S, Wacker KM. (2020) The rise of robots and the fall of routine jobs. *Labour Economics*, **66**(2020), 101885.
14. Birnbaum B. (2019) The rise of human agents: AI-powered customer service automation. https://www.forbes.com/sites/bradbirnbaum/2019/06/19/the-rise-of-human-agents-ai-powered-customer-service-automation/?sh=684fba8793f2 accessed 8/16/23

15. Go H. (2022) Digital pathology and artificial intelligence applications in pathology. *Brain Tumor Research and Treatment*, **10**(2), 76–82.

16. Jadczyk T, Wojakowski W, Tendera M, Henry TD, Egnaczyk G, Shreenivas S. (2021) Artificial intelligence can improve patient management at the time of a pandemic: the role of voice technology. *Journal of Medical Internet Research*, **23**(5), e22959.

17. (2023) The benefits of AI-enabled virtual nursing assistants. https://artificialintelligenceinnursing.com/the-benefits-of-ai-enabled-virtual-nursing-assistants/

18. Brand JE. (2015) The far-reaching impact of job loss and unemployment. *Annual Review of Sociology*, **41**, 359–375.

19. Jha S, Topol EJ. (2016) Adapting to artificial intelligence: radiologists and pathologists as information specialists. *JAMA Network*, **316**(22), 2353–2354.

20. Shortliffe EH, Sepúlveda MJ. (2018) Clinical decision support in the era of artificial intelligence. *JAMA Network*, **320**(21), 2199–2200.

Chapter 11

AI Tools and Applications in Clinical Practice

Introduction

AI tools and applications have the potential to significantly impact clinical practice, improving patient care, enhancing efficiency, and supporting clinical decision-making. From diagnostic support to treatment recommendations, risk assessment, and patient monitoring, AI can augment the capabilities of healthcare professionals. In this chapter, we will provide an overview of AI tools and applications used in clinical practice, discuss their benefits in improving patient care and enhancing efficiency, and address potential concerns associated with AI in healthcare.

Overview of AI tools and applications used in clinical practice

AI encompasses a variety of technologies and techniques that enable machines to perform tasks that typically require human intelligence. In the medical field, AI tools and applications are used to analyze large datasets, extract meaningful insights, and support clinical decision-making. These tools include machine learning algorithms, natural language processing, computer vision, and robotics.

Types of AI tools and applications in clinical practice

AI is utilized in various areas of clinical practice to improve patient care and support healthcare professionals. In diagnostic support, AI algorithms can analyze medical images, such as retinal fundus photographs, to detect conditions like diabetic retinopathy.[1] AI has also shown promise in dermatology, where deep neural networks achieve a dermatologist-level classification of skin cancer. Moreover, AI algorithms can assist in the interpretation of chest radiographs and detect arrhythmias in electrocardiograms, aiding in diagnosis and treatment planning.

Real-world examples of AI tools being used in clinics include:

- Diagnostic imaging: AI algorithms have demonstrated excellent accuracy in the detection of small radiographic abnormalities, assisting radiologists in identifying and quantifying various clinical conditions. In a recent study published in Nature Communication, researchers at Emory University focused on utilizing a deep learning model to detect type 2 diabetes (T2D) by combining radiographic and electronic health records (EHR) data.[2] The model was trained using a dataset consisting of 271,065 ambulatory chest radiographs (CXRs) from 160,244 unique patients. To evaluate its performance, the model was tested on a prospective dataset containing 9,943 CXRs. The results revealed that the deep learning model effectively detected T2D, achieving a receiver operating characteristic area under the curve (ROC AUC) of 0.84, with a prevalence of 16%. Notably, the algorithm identified 1,381 cases (14%) as suspicious for T2D. External validation conducted at a different institution yielded a ROC AUC of 0.77, and subsequently, 5% of patients were diagnosed with T2D. Furthermore, the researchers employed explainable AI techniques to identify correlations between specific adiposity measures and high predictivity. As CXRs are common and relatively inexpensive tests, this study highlights the potential of CXRs in enhancing T2D screening. There are many non-interpretive problems that AI is solving in radiology departments today. For example, AI programs optimize image acquisition and reconstruction by improving the signal-to-noise ratio in MRI scans.[3,4] These programs allow faster scan times without sacrificing image quality. Other deep learning tools can reconstruct high-quality images from low-dose CT or PET data, reducing the usual high radiation doses usually associated with creating high-quality images.[5]

- Laboratory medicine: AI has been applied to improve the value and efficiency of laboratory testing, including automating test result interpretation, optimizing workflow, and predicting disease outcomes.[6,7] It has shown promise in predicting disease outcomes based on laboratory data.[8] By analyzing a patient's laboratory test results along with other clinical data, AI models can generate predictive models that estimate the likelihood of disease progression, response to treatment, or the risk of developing complications. These predictive models can assist healthcare providers in making informed decisions regarding patient management and treatment strategies.

- Patient safety: Although more than twenty years have elapsed since the Institute of Medicine's "To Err Is Human" report,[9] patient safety problems remain all too common.[10] In fact, according to a recent study by researchers at Johns Hopkins University, an estimated 161,000 preventable deaths occur in the U.S. each year based on the most current data available.[11] AI holds the potential to improve patient safety by predicting, preventing, or detecting adverse events across various domains, such as healthcare-associated infections, adverse drug events, surgical complications, and diagnostic errors.[12] AI has been used to analyze the data from multiple patient sensing technologies including vital sign monitoring, wearables, pressure sensors, and computer vision, and to alert the healthcare team when dangerous situations arise.

- Clinical decision support: AI-based clinical decision support tools are used to augment healthcare professionals in making complex evidence-based treatment recommendations, medication management, and mental health support.[13,14] Using AI-powered clinical decision support systems in healthcare can lead to better quality of care, more appropriate use of healthcare resources, and less provider burnout. These tools are now commonly accessed through electronic medical record systems.

These examples highlight the wide-ranging applications of AI in clinical practice, demonstrating its potential to improve accuracy, efficiency, and patient outcomes. As AI continues to evolve, it can transform healthcare delivery and support healthcare professionals in providing optimal care to their patients.

Benefits of AI in clinical practice

The integration of AI in clinical practice offers numerous benefits. AI tools can enhance the accuracy and efficiency of diagnoses, leading to improved patient outcomes.[15] By analyzing patient data and medical records, AI algorithms can provide treatment recommendations tailored to individual patients, thereby supporting personalized medicine.[16] AI also enables risk assessment by identifying high-risk individuals, predicting disease progression, and aiding in the early detection of diseases. Furthermore, AI-powered patient monitoring systems facilitate continuous remote monitoring, enabling timely interventions and better disease management.

Addressing concerns associated with AI in healthcare

While AI holds great promise in medicine, it is essential to address concerns associated with its implementation. Privacy and security of patient data are critical considerations.[17] Hence, it is crucial to ensure proper data governance and comply with relevant regulations to protect patient privacy. The lack of transparency and interpretability of AI algorithms is another concern. Researchers are developing explainable AI models that can provide clinicians with insights into the decision-making process of AI systems. Additionally, addressing the potential biases in AI algorithms and ensuring equitable access to AI-based healthcare solutions are important considerations.

Diagnostic support

AI algorithms have a significant role in diagnostic support, aiding physicians in accurate and timely diagnoses across various medical specialties.

The integration of AI enhances diagnostic accuracy, improves efficiency, and enables personalized treatment recommendations.

Role of AI in diagnostic support

AI algorithms play a vital role in diagnostic support, particularly in image recognition and analysis. By utilizing advanced computer vision techniques, AI algorithms can analyze medical images such as X-rays, CT scans, and mammograms.[18] This capability enables them to detect subtle abnormalities and provide valuable insights to assist physicians in making accurate diagnoses. Additionally, AI algorithms excel in pattern recognition, allowing them to identify complex relationships within large datasets. By learning from extensive medical data, AI algorithms can detect patterns that may not be easily discernible to human observers, such as the fat distribution in chest X-rays that can be used to screen for diabetes noted in the section above. This enables physicians to identify risk factors, predict disease progression, and make personalized treatment recommendations, improving patient outcomes.

Benefits of AI in diagnostic support

Diagnostic errors are frequent and often result in death or disability.[19] Indeed, in the USA, more than a million people per year are harmed by diagnostic errors.[20] According to a report from the U.S. Institute of Medicine at the National Academies of Science, Engineering, and Medicine (NASEM), diagnostic errors contribute to approximately 10% of patient deaths and account for 6% to 17% of hospital complications.[21] However, these errors are typically not caused by outright physician negligence but rather a combination of factors including human error, inefficient collaboration between organizations, and communication gaps among caregivers.

The impact of diagnostic mistakes is significant, both in terms of patient harm and financial costs. A review conducted by Johns Hopkins revealed that the total payout attributed to diagnostic errors in the U.S. amount to approximately $100 million a year.[22] Thus, it is evident that there is room for improvement in current diagnostic and treatment standards. Recognizing the prevalence and impact of diagnostic errors is crucial for driving change and enhancing patient safety. One of the ways to decrease these errors is through the integration of AI systems into clinical medicine.

The integration of AI in diagnostic support brings numerous benefits to physicians and patients. AI algorithms enhance diagnostic accuracy by reducing errors associated with human interpretation and judgment. According to a 2020 study in The Lancet by Oren, *et al.*, AI systems used in medical imaging can achieve comparable or even superior performance to human experts in various diagnostic tasks, reducing misdiagnoses and improving patient outcomes.[23]

AI algorithms can also significantly improve the efficiency of the diagnostic process.[24] They can rapidly analyze vast amounts of patient data, identify relevant patterns, and generate preliminary diagnoses. This allows physicians to focus on critical cases and make timely treatment decisions. According to an article written by Maryann Hardy, published in the 2020 British Journal of Radiology, AI-powered tools also have the potential to alleviate the workload burden on healthcare professionals by automating routine tasks, enabling them to allocate more time to direct patient care.[25]

Examples of AI tools in diagnostic support

AI tools are extensively used in various medical specialties to aid in diagnostic support. In radiology, AI algorithms assist in the detection of abnormalities in medical images, such as lung nodules, fractures, and breast lesions. Ohad Oren opines in a 2020 Lancet article on AI in medical imaging, "AI might identify imaging pattern changes that are not easily amenable to human identification.[23] For example, acute management of ischemic stroke is dependent on a prompt diagnosis. Current ischemic stroke guidelines state that patients are eligible for intravenous thrombolysis up to 4.5 hours from symptom onset and endovascular thrombectomy within 6 hours of symptom onset.[26] However, ischemic changes are often not appreciated by radiologists that soon after the event. An analysis of brain MRIs using machine learning has the potential to identify tissue changes reflective of early ischemic stroke within the narrow time window from symptom onset with greater sensitivity than a human reader."[27]

New research from the University of California San Diego School of Medicine has demonstrated the potential of AI in differentiating between Kawasaki disease and multisystem inflammatory syndrome in children (MIS-C).[28] Led by Jane Burns, the team developed an AI model called KIDMATCH to aid clinicians in distinguishing between these two conditions using test results and physical examination features. The study followed a two-stage process. Firstly, the researchers enrolled 1,538 children with MIS-C or a diagnosis of Kawasaki disease for internal validation. The KIDMATCH AI model was trained to differentiate MIS-C from other pediatric febrile illnesses. The researchers developed a deep-learning system that utilized data such as the patient's age, the five classic clinical signs of Kawasaki's disease, and 17 laboratory studies to suggest a diagnosis. Subsequently, the model was trained to differentiate Kawasaki disease from other pediatric febrile conditions. During internal validation, the AI model achieved a median area under the receiver operating characteristic curve of 98.8% in stage one and 96.0% in stage two. In external validation, the model successfully identified MIS-C in 94% of cases. These results are promising and highlight the potential of AI models like KIDMATCH in aiding clinicians in the differentiation of Kawasaki disease and MIS-C, as well as other pediatric febrile illnesses.

By implementing AI models like KIDMATCH, earlier detection of diseases can be achieved, leading to timely interventions, prevention of complications, and improved patient outcomes. This research marks a significant advancement, especially considering that creating a diagnostic test for Kawasaki disease has been a challenge for the Kawasaki research community for the past 40 years. The use of AI in disease-specific pathways has the potential to enhance healthcare by improving diagnostic accuracy and facilitating early intervention.

Another example of an AI system improving accuracy is in the diagnosis of acute myocardial infarction. Despite appropriate testing of chest pain patients, the diagnosis can often be missed. Approximately 30% of patients with an occluded coronary artery do not have the characteristic EKG findings of elevated ST segments,[29] and 25% of patients subsequently diagnosed with acute MI do not have elevated high-sensitivity troponin levels.[30] This results in a delayed diagnosis of 25% to 30% of patients with acute MI. These patients often miss the opportunity for reperfusion therapy and can have a poor prognosis. The researcher Al-Zaiti and colleagues at the University of Pittsburgh published an article in Nature Medicine that addressed this issue.[31] They evaluated 7,313 patients with acute chest pain, feeding their EKG results and electronic medical records into an AI system. The results demonstrated that the AI-derived risk score successfully reclassified one-third of the patients, that is, the AI system identified one-third of the patients with negative EKG findings as having an acute MI. This surpassed the performance of both clinical experts and commercial ECG interpretation systems. Moreover, the study prioritized the transparency and interpretability of the model by identifying the 25 most influential features of the EKG that drove its accuracy. The researchers summarized their findings as follows, "This study represents the first use of machine learning techniques and novel ECG features to optimize the detection of occlusive myocardial infarction in patients presenting with acute chest pain and negative ST-elevation myocardial infarction (STEMI) patterns on their initial ECG."

AI also plays an important role in the field of pathology, where computational pathology algorithms analyze histopathological images. These algorithms assist pathologists in diagnosing diseases, including cancer, by identifying patterns and features that may not be easily discernible to the human eye. This improves diagnostic accuracy and enables personalized treatment recommendations. An example of this use of AI to improve the accuracy of pathologic diagnosis and provide treatment recommendations is a company called PreciseDx. AI-driven platforms like PreciseDx are transforming the field of pathology and personalized treatment recommendations. PreciseDx, a New York City-based company, has developed an innovative AI platform that leverages AI to enhance the accuracy of pathologic diagnosis and provide personalized treatment recommendations for breast and prostate tissue biopsies.[32] By analyzing millions of data points, the PreciseDx platform captures a wealth of information from each slide, stain, and tissue sample, surpassing what is humanly possible. Through this AI-driven analysis, the platform identifies a set of 8 to 12 disease-specific key features, enabling standardized grading and a risk stratification score that indicates patient risk and offers valuable insights for potential treatment approaches.

The use of standardized, quantitative metrics and AI in the PreciseDx platform significantly improves diagnostic accuracy and enables tailored treatment recommendations. Pathologists and oncologists can use the platform's insights and actionable intelligence to create the most effective treatment for each patient. This AI platform provides highly accurate risk profiles, enhances diagnostic precision, reduces error rates, and ultimately contributes to improved patient outcomes while decreasing costs.

Limitations and challenges of solely relying on AI for diagnosis

While AI brings significant advancements to diagnostic support, there are limitations and challenges to relying solely on AI for diagnosis. One limitation is the need for high-quality and diverse training data. AI algorithms rely heavily on well-curated datasets for training and the availability of such datasets can be a challenge, particularly for rare diseases or specific patient populations. Interpreting and understanding the decisions made by AI algorithms, often referred to as the "black box" problem, is another challenge. AI algorithms can provide accurate predictions, but the underlying reasoning and explanation may not always be transparent to physicians. Ensuring the interpretability and explainability of AI algorithms is essential for establishing trust and acceptance among physicians. Moreover, relying solely on AI for diagnosis raises ethical considerations. Physicians must balance the benefits of AI with patient autonomy, privacy, and the potential for overreliance on AI systems. It is crucial to maintain a human-in-the-loop approach, where AI algorithms serve as decision support tools rather than replacing the clinical expertise and judgment of physicians.

AI algorithms have a significant role in diagnostic support, aiding physicians in accurate and timely diagnoses across various medical specialties. The integration of AI enhances diagnostic accuracy, improves efficiency, enables personalized treatment recommendations, and decreases clinical errors. However, it is important to recognize the limitations and challenges of relying solely on AI for diagnosis, including the need for high-quality training data, interpretability of AI algorithms, and ethical considerations. By embracing a collaborative approach that combines the strengths of AI with the clinical expertise of physicians, we can unlock the full potential of AI in improving healthcare outcomes.

Treatment recommendation

The use of AI in treatment recommendation and personalized medicine holds great potential for transforming healthcare delivery. AI algorithms can leverage patient data, medical records, and clinical guidelines to generate tailored treatment recommendations, optimizing therapeutic interventions and improving patient outcomes. This section explores the application of AI in treatment recommendation, highlighting its potential to optimize treatment plans and enhance patient outcomes. Case studies showcasing successful AI implementation in treatment recommendations will be presented to illustrate real-world examples.

AI algorithms for analyzing patient data

AI algorithms play a vital role in the analysis of patient data, enabling healthcare providers to extract meaningful insights and make informed treatment recommendations.[24] Machine learning techniques, such as supervised learning and deep learning, are applied to large datasets, allowing algorithms to identify patterns, associations, and correlations within the data. This analysis includes factors such as patient demographics, medical history, genetic information, and treatment outcomes. By considering these multifaceted data points, AI algorithms can generate personalized treatment recommendations based on the unique characteristics of each patient.

Utilizing medical records and clinical guidelines

Medical records contain a wealth of valuable information about patients, including diagnoses, medications, laboratory results, and imaging reports. AI algorithms can process and analyze these records to uncover patterns and extract relevant information, providing a comprehensive understanding of a patient's medical history. Additionally, AI algorithms can integrate clinical guidelines, which are evidence-based recommendations for specific medical conditions, into their decision-making process. By aligning patient data with established clinical guidelines, AI algorithms can suggest treatment options that are consistent with best practices and the most up-to-date medical knowledge.

Optimizing treatment plans with AI

One of the significant advantages of AI in treatment recommendation is its ability to optimize treatment plans based on individual patient characteristics. According to estimates from the research firm Frost & Sullivan, the use of AI has the potential to increase positive patient outcomes by 30% to 40% while decreasing treatment costs by up to 50%.[34] AI algorithms consider various factors, including patient demographics, genetic predispositions, treatment response data, and clinical guidelines, to generate personalized treatment recommendations. These recommendations can help physicians select the most effective interventions, minimize adverse reactions, and tailor therapies to meet the specific needs of each patient. These AI systems can also identify patients who are unlikely to benefit from medical treatment or surgical procedures. This can save time, money, and resources for both patients and the healthcare system. By leveraging AI, treatment plans can be continuously refined and adjusted based on real-time patient data, leading to improved outcomes and enhanced patient satisfaction.

Case studies of successful AI implementation

Several case studies demonstrate the successful implementation of AI in treatment recommendations. For example, in oncology, AI algorithms have been employed to analyze genomic data, identify genetic markers associated with specific tumors, and suggest targeted therapies tailored to individual patients.[35] This approach has shown promising results in improving treatment outcomes and survival rates. In another case, AI algorithms have been used to analyze patient data in mental health conditions and recommend personalized treatment plans, such as medication selection and dosage optimization, leading to enhanced symptom management and patient well-being.[36,37]

Risk assessment

AI has emerged as a powerful tool in healthcare, revolutionizing risk assessment, early disease detection, and identification of high-risk individuals. By providing valuable insights, AI systems can aid in accurate risk assessment and prediction.

Risk assessment and prediction models

Risk assessment is the process of identifying what potential hazards exist or may occur in any projected activity or undertaking. In healthcare, it plays a vital role in identifying individuals susceptible to diseases or adverse events. AI offers several advantages in risk assessment and prediction models. With its ability to process large volumes of patient data, identify patterns and trends, and generate accurate predictions, AI enhances risk assessment accuracy. Furthermore, AI systems continuously adapt and learn from new data, improving performance over time. One example of the AI risk assessment model includes Predictive OpTimal Trees in Emergency Surgery Risk (POTTER), developed by the Center for Outcomes & Patient Safety in Surgery (COMPASS), which utilizes AI to predict and model surgical risks and determine the best interventions for high-risk patients.[38] Another example is Mirai, an AI tool developed by scientists from MIT's Computer Science and Artificial Intelligence Laboratory (CSAIL) and Jameel Clinic, designed to predict cancer risk using a patient's mammogram.[39] Clinical risk factors such as age, lifestyle, or family history are used to model a patient's risk across multiple future time points by the deep learning system.

Utilization of machine learning algorithms

Machine learning algorithms empower AI systems to analyze patient data and identify risk factors. These algorithms uncover complex relationships and patterns, leading to more accurate risk assessment and prediction. Various machine learning algorithms, including supervised learning, unsupervised learning, and reinforcement learning, contribute to risk assessment. As was mentioned in earlier chapters, supervised learning algorithms learn from labeled data, unsupervised learning algorithms identify patterns in unlabeled data, and reinforcement learning algorithms optimize decisions based on feedback.

AI for early disease detection

Early disease detection significantly improves patient outcomes and treatment effectiveness. AI systems analyze patient data, identify subtle patterns, and provide timely alerts to healthcare providers, facilitating early disease detection.[39,40] AI has proven successful in early disease detection across multiple areas. For instance, AI algorithms analyze medical imaging data to detect early signs of cancer, identify subtle abnormalities in electrocardiogram (ECG) patterns indicative of heart conditions, and analyze biomarkers for early detection of neurological disorders. An example of this is seen in an article in the edition of Nature Medicine on May 8th, 2023.[41] It reported that researchers at Harvard Medical School and the University of Copenhagen had been able to identify people with the highest risk of pancreatic cancer up to three years before the actual diagnosis by employing an AI program to review their medical records. The AI algorithm was trained on two separate data sets totaling 9 million patient records from Denmark and the United States. The researchers used the AI model to identify risk factors based on the data contained in the records. The model was able to predict which patients are likely to develop pancreatic cancer in the future based on risks found in the medical record such as a family history of pancreatic cancer, a history of gall bladder disease, and diabetes, among others. The researchers said they believe the model is at least as accurate in predicting disease occurrence as are current genetic sequencing tests. These genetic tests are usually available only for a small subset of patients. Screening software like this could be embedded into ERHs allowing healthcare professionals to send high-risk patients for CT scans or other screening methodologies.

Prediction of adverse events

AI contributes to predictive models that identify patients at risk of adverse events such as hospital-acquired infections, medication errors, or surgical complications.[42,43] By analyzing patient data, AI systems can flag high-risk individuals, thereby enabling proactive interventions. Real-world applications demonstrate the effectiveness of AI in predicting adverse events. For instance, AI algorithms analyze EHRs to identify patients at risk of sepsis, predict falls in hospitalized patients based on sensor data, and detect medication errors through natural language processing techniques.[44,45] AI frameworks have also been used to evaluate carotid ultrasound for predictive cardiovascular and stroke risk assessment.[46]

Identification of high-risk individuals

Accurate identification of high-risk individuals allows for targeted interventions, preventive measures, and personalized treatment plans. AI contributes to risk stratification models that effectively identify high-risk individuals.[47] AI algorithms analyze diverse patient data sources, including EHRs, genetic data, lifestyle factors, and social determinants of health, to identify high-risk individuals. For example, AI can help identify individuals at high risk of developing cardiovascular diseases, diabetes, or mental health conditions.[48,49] This is especially helpful in patients who present with a medical problem that can distract the healthcare team from other serious underlying health risks.

Patient monitoring

The role of continuous AI monitoring of patients in healthcare is a transformative aspect that enhances remote healthcare and patient management.

Continuous patient monitoring and remote healthcare

Continuous patient monitoring is revolutionized by AI, enabling remote healthcare delivery, and improving patient care. AI can be applied to remote patient monitoring (RPM), which utilizes wearable devices,

Internet of Things (IoT) methodologies, and telehealth applications.[50,51] RPM is now a common healthcare methodology for monitoring patients with acute or chronic illnesses in the hospital or remote locations. This monitoring can occur over various domains, including chronic disease management programs, post-operative care, and general wellness.

It encompasses the measurement of vital signs and other physiological parameters through wearable biosensors, providing clinicians with real-time data to support clinical judgments and treatment plans. Wearable biosensors typically are non-invasive devices used to acquire, transmit, process, store, and retrieve health-related data including heart rate, respiration, blood oxygenation, and serum glucose levels. These biosensors have been integrated into watches, wristbands, skin patches, shoes, belts, textiles, and smartphones. The incorporation of AI into these RPM systems enhances their capabilities and enables proactive monitoring, early detection of health issues, and improved patient outcomes.[52]

Benefits of AI-based patient monitoring

AI-based patient monitoring offers numerous advantages in healthcare.[53] By leveraging AI algorithms, continuous monitoring systems can analyze patient data in real-time, detect patterns, and provide actionable insights. For instance, AI enables personalized monitoring and intervention strategies for chronic diseases, facilitating timely interventions and reducing hospital readmissions.

Conclusion

AI tools and applications have significantly impacted clinical practice, offering benefits in diagnostic support, treatment recommendation, risk assessment, and patient monitoring. These advancements have the potential to improve patient care, enhance efficiency, and support healthcare professionals in providing optimal care to their patients. By addressing concerns and embracing a collaborative approach, AI can transform healthcare delivery and improve healthcare outcomes.

References

1. Padhy SK, Takkar B, Chawla R, Kumar A. (2019) Artificial intelligence in diabetic retinopathy: a natural step to the future. *Indian Journal of Ophthalmology*, **67**(7), 1004–1009.

2. Pyrros A, Borstelmann SM, Mantravadi R, *et al.* (2023) Opportunistic detection of type 2 diabetes using deep learning from frontal chest radiographs. *Nature Communications*, **14**, 4039.

3. Blum K. (2023) A status report on AI in laboratory medicine. https://www.aacc.org/cln/articles/2023/janfeb/a-status-report-on-ai-in-laboratory-medicine

4. Lin DJ, Johnson PM, Knoll F, Lui YW. (2021) Artificial intelligence for MR image reconstruction: an overview for clinicians. *Journal of Magnetic Resonance Imaging*, **53**, 1015–1028.

5. Yaqub M, Jinchao F, Arshid K, Ahmed S, Zhang W, Nawaz MZ, Mahmood T. (2022) Deep learning-based image reconstruction for different medical imaging modalities. *Computational and Mathematical Methods in Medicine*, **2022**, 8750648.

6. Rabbani N, Kim GYE, Suarez CJ, Chen JH. (2022) Applications of machine learning in routine laboratory medicine: current state and future directions. *Clinical Biochemistry*, **103,** 1–7.

7. Ahmad Z, Rahim S, Zubair M, Abdul-Ghafar J. (2021) Artificial intelligence (AI) in medicine, current applications and future role with special emphasis on its potential and promise in pathology: present and future impact, obstacles including costs and acceptance among pathologists, practical and philosophical considerations. A comprehensive review. *Diagnostic Pathology*, **16**(1), 24.

8. Kumar Y, Koul A, Singla R, Ijaz MF. (2023) Artificial intelligence in disease diagnosis: a systematic literature review, synthesizing framework and future research agenda. *Journal of Ambient Intelligence and Humanized Computing*, **14**(7), 8459–8486.

9. Kohn LT, Corrigan JM, Donaldson MS, Institute of Medicine (US) Committee on Quality of Health Care in America. (2000) To Err is Human: Building a Safer Health System. *National Academies Press (US)*, PMID: 25077248.

10. Wilensky GR. (2019) Patient safety issues continue to plague American hospitals. *The Milbank Quarterly*, **97**(3):641–644.

11. Austin M, Derek J. (2019) Lives lost, lives saved: an updated comparative analysis of avoidable deaths at hospitals graded by the Leapfrog Group. Armstrong Institute for Patient Safety and Quality, Johns Hopkins Medicine. https://www.hospitalsafetygrade.org/media/file/Lives-Saved-White-Paper-FINAL.pdf

12. Bates DW, Levine D, Syrowatka A, *et al.* (2021) The potential of artificial intelligence to improve patient safety: a scoping review. *npj Digital Medicine*, **4**, 54.

13. Bajgain B, Lorenzetti D, Lee J, *et al.* (2023) Determinants of implementing artificial intelligence-based clinical decision support tools in healthcare: a scoping review protocol. *BMJ Open*, **13**, e068373.

14. Sutton RT, Pincock D, Baumgart DC, *et al.* (2020) An overview of clinical decision support systems: benefits, risks, and strategies for success. *npj Digital Medicine*, **3**, 17.

15. Al-Antari MA. (2023) Artificial Intelligence for Medical Diagnostics-Existing and Future AI Technology! *Diagnostics (Basel)*, **13**(4), 688.

16. Schork NJ. (2019) Artificial intelligence and personalized medicine. *Cancer Treatment Research*, **178**, 265–283.

17. Murdoch B. (2021) Privacy and artificial intelligence: challenges for protecting health information in a new era. *BMC Med Ethics*, **22**, 122.

18. Hosny A, Parmar C, Quackenbush J, Schwartz LH, Aerts HJWL. (2018) Artificial intelligence in radiology. *Nature Reviews Cancer*, **18**(8), 500–510.

19. Graber ML. (2013) The incidence of diagnostic error in medicine. *BMJ Quality & Safety*, **22** Suppl 2(Suppl 2), ii21–ii27.

20. Newman-Toker DE, Makary MA. (2013) Measuring diagnostic errors in primary care: the first step on a path forward. Comment on "Types and origins of diagnostic errors in primary care settings". *JAMA Internal Medicine*, **173**, 425–426.

21. Balogh EP, Miller BT, Ball JR, Committee on Diagnostic Error in Health Care, Board on Health Care Services, Institute of Medicine, The National Academies of Sciences, Engineering, and Medicine. (2015) Improving diagnosis in health care. *National Academies Press (US)*, PMID: 26803862.

22. Newman-Toker DE. (2015) Diagnostic value: the economics of high-quality diagnosis and a value-based perspective on diagnostic innovation. In *Modern Healthcare Annual Patient Safety & Quality Virtual Conference*.

23. Oren O, Gersh BJ, Bhatt DL. (2020) Artificial intelligence in medical imaging: switching from radiographic pathological data to clinically meaningful endpoints. *The Lancet Digital Health*, **2**(9), e486–e488.
24. Dave M, Patel N. (2023) Artificial intelligence in healthcare and education. *British Dental Journal*, **234**, 761–764 (2023).
25. Hardy M, Harvey H. (2020) Artificial intelligence in diagnostic imaging: impact on the radiography profession. *The British Journal of Radiology*, **93**(1108), 20190840.
26. Powers WJ, Rabinstein AA, Ackerson T, Adeoye OM, Bambakidis NC, Becker K, *et al.* (2018) 2018 Guidelines for the early management of patients with acute ischemic stroke: a guideline for healthcare professionals from the American Heart Association/American Stroke Association. *Stroke*, **49**, e46–e110.
27. Gauriau R, Bizzo BC, Comeau DS, *et al.* (2023) Head CT deep learning model is highly accurate for early infarct estimation. *Scientific Reports*, **13**, 189.
28. Lam JY, Shimizu C, Tremoulet AH, Bainto E, Roberts SC, Sivilay N, Gardiner MA, Kanegaye JT, Hogan AH, Salazar JC, Mohandas S, Szmuszkovicz JR, Mahanta S, Dionne A, Newburger JW, Ansusinha E, DeBiasi RL, Hao S, Ling XB, Cohen HJ, Nemati S, Burns JC, Pediatric Emergency Medicine Kawasaki Disease Research Group, CHARMS Study Group. (2022) A machine-learning algorithm for diagnosis of multisystem inflammatory syndrome in children and Kawasaki disease in the USA: a retrospective model development and validation study. *The Lancet Digital Health*, **4**(10), e717–e726.
29. Sharma M, Khanal RR, Shah S, Gajurel RM, Poudel CM, Adhikari S, Yadav V, Devkota S, Thapa S. (2023) Occluded coronary artery among non-ST elevation myocardial infarction patients in department of cardiology of a tertiary care centre: a descriptive cross-sectional study. *Journal of Nepal Medical Association*, **61**(257), 54–58.
30. Body R, Carley S, McDowell G, Jaffe AS, France M, Cruickshank K, *et al.* (2011) Rapid exclusion of acute myocardial infarction in patients with undetectable troponin using a high-sensitivity assay. *Journal of the American College of Cardiology*, **58**, 1332–1339.
31. Al-Zaiti SS, Martin-Gill C, Zègre-Hemsey JK, *et al.* (2023) Machine learning for ECG diagnosis and risk stratification of occlusion myocardial infarction. *Nature Medicine*, **29**, 1804–1813.
32. Fernandez G, Prastawa M, Madduri AS, Scott R, Marami B, Shpalensky N, Cascetta K, Sawyer M, Chan M, Koll G, Shtabsky A, Feliz A, Hansen T,

Veremis B, Cordon-Cardo C, Zeineh J, Donovan MJ. (2022) Development and validation of an AI-enabled digital breast cancer assay to predict early-stage breast cancer recurrence within 6 years. *Breast Cancer Research,* **24**(1), 93.

33. Price WN. (2019) Risks and remedies for artificial intelligence in health care. https://www.brookings.edu/articles/risks-and-remedies-for-artificial-intelligence-in-health-care/

34. Hsieh P (2017) AI in medicine: rise of the machines. https://www.forbes.com/sites/paulhsieh/2017/04/30/ai-in-medicine-rise-of-the-machines/

35. Liao J, Li X, Gan Y, Han S, Rong P, Wang W, Li W, Zhou L. (2023) Artificial intelligence assists precision medicine in cancer treatment. *Frontiers in Oncology,* **12**, 998222.

36. Graham S, Depp C, Lee EE, Nebeker C, Tu X, Kim HC, Jeste DV. (2019) Artificial intelligence for mental health and mental illnesses: an overview. Current Psychiatry Reports, **21**(11), 116.

37. Mahdieh Montazeri, *et al.* (2022) Application of machine learning methods in predicting schizophrenia and bipolar disorders: a systematic review. *Health Science Reports,* **6**(1), e962.

38. El Hechi MW, Maurer LR, Levine J, Zhuo D, El Moheb M, Velmahos GC, Dunn J, Bertsimas D, Kaafarani HM. (2021) Validation of the Artificial Intelligence-Based Predictive Optimal Trees in Emergency Surgery Risk (POTTER) calculator in emergency general surgery and emergency laparotomy patients. *Journal of the American College of Surgeons,* **232**(6), 912–919.

39. Gordon R. (2021) Robust artificial intelligence tools to predict future cancer. https://news.mit.edu/2021/robust-artificial-intelligence-tools-predict-future-cancer-0128

40. Kourou K, *et al.* (2015) Machine learning applications in cancer prognosis and prediction. *Computational and Structural Biotechnology Journal,* **13**, 8–17.

41. Miotto R, Li L, Kidd B, *et al.* (2016) Deep patient: an unsupervised representation to predict the future of patients from the electronic health records. *Scientific Reports,* **6**, 26094.

42. Veldhuis LI, Woittiez NJC, Nanayakkara PWB, Ludikhuize J. (2022) Artificial Intelligence for the prediction of in-hospital clinical deterioration: a systematic review. *Critical Care Explorations,* **4**(9), e0744.

43. Choudhury A, Asan O. (2020) Role of artificial intelligence in patient safety outcomes: systematic literature review. *JMIR Medical Informatics,* **8**(7), e18599.

44. Macias CG, Remy KE, Barda AJ. Utilizing big data from electronic health records in pediatric clinical care. Pediatr Res. 2023 Jan;93(2):382–389. doi:

10.1038/s41390-022-02343-x. Epub 2022 Nov 24. PMID: 36434202; PMCID: PMC9702658.

45. Bates DW, Levine D, Syrowatka A, *et al.* (2021) The potential of artificial intelligence to improve patient safety: a scoping review. *npj Digital. Medicine*, **4**, 54 (2021).

46. Jamthikar AD, Gupta D, Saba L, Khanna NN, Viskovic K, Mavrogeni S, Laird JR, Sattar N, Johri AM, Pareek G, Miner M, Sfikakis PP, Protogerou A, Viswanathan V, Sharma A, Kitas GD, Nicolaides A, Kolluri R, Suri JS. (2020) Artificial intelligence framework for predictive cardiovascular and stroke risk assessment models: A narrative review of integrated approaches using carotid ultrasound. *Computers in Biology and Medicine*, **126**:104043.

47. Carroll N, Jones A. (2022) Improving risk stratification using ai and social determinants of health. *The American Journal of Managed Care*, **28**(11), 582–587.

48. Weiss JC, Natarajan S, Peissig PL, McCarty CA, Page D. (2012) Machine learning for personalized medicine: predicting primary myocardial infarction from electronic health records. *AI Magazine: Home of AI and Artificial Intelligence News,* **33**, 33.

49. Pereira-Morales AJ, Rojas LH. (2022) Risk stratification using Artificial Intelligence: Could it be useful to reduce the burden of chronic kidney disease in low- and middle-income Countries? *Frontiers in Public Health*, **10**, 999512.

50. Alshamrani M. (2022) IoT and artificial intelligence implementations for remote healthcare monitoring systems: a survey. *Journal of King Saud University — Computer and Information Sciences*, **34**(8), 4687–4701.

51. Ahila A, Dahan F, Alroobaea R, Alghamdi WY, Mustafa Khaja Mohammed, Hajjej F, Deema Mohammed Alsekait, Raahemifar K. (2023) A smart IoMT based architecture for E-healthcare patient monitoring system using artificial intelligence algorithms. Frontiers in Physiology, **14**, 1125952.

52. Farid F, Bello A, Ahamed F, Hossain F. (2023) The roles of AI technologies in reducing hospital readmission for chronic diseases: a comprehensive analysis. Preprints 2023, 2023071000. https://doi.org/10.20944/pre-prints202307.1000.v1

53. Lu ZX, Qian P, Bi D, Ye ZW, He X, Zhao YH, Su L, Li SL, Zhu ZL. (2021) Application of AI and IoT in clinical medicine: summary and challenges. *Current Medical Science*, **41**, 1134–1150.

Chapter 12

Implementing AI in Clinical Settings

Introduction

The implementation of artificial intelligence (AI) in clinical settings holds great promise for transforming healthcare delivery. However, it also presents unique challenges and considerations that need to be addressed for successful integration. This chapter focuses on the practical aspects of implementing AI in clinical settings, discussing the challenges, considerations, and strategies for healthcare professionals to effectively incorporate AI technologies into their workflow.

Assessing organizational readiness

Successfully integrating AI into clinical workflows requires careful assessment of an organization's readiness. Healthcare leaders should conduct an objective analysis of their current data infrastructure, workflows, and processes to identify strengths, weaknesses, opportunities, and threats with respect to AI adoption.

A readiness assessment should evaluate several key areas. One is clinical workflows, which involves mapping out current care pathways and processes, looking for bottlenecks, redundancies, or places where AI could provide automation, prediction, or decision support. It is also important to assess clinician openness to adapting workflows. The successful integration of AI into clinical settings depends heavily on frontline clinician adoption and utilization. If clinicians are resistant to changing workflows or mistrust new technologies, then AI initiatives will likely fail or underperform. As such, assessing clinician attitudes and openness to workflow changes is a critical component of evaluating organizational readiness for AI.

This assessment can be done through surveys, focus groups, and informal interviews with physicians, nurses, and other staff who will be impacted by AI implementation. This information gathering should include the following steps: catalog existing data sources, formats, and systems, evaluating the quality, completeness, and accessibility of data. Determine abilities to link disparate data and identify any limitations or gaps in infrastructure. Document existing IT systems and integration capabilities and assess readiness to deploy new AI within the current ecosystem. Identify clinical areas, operations, or tasks that could benefit from AI to focus on for pilot opportunities.

Finally, evaluate organizational culture — the willingness to adopt new technologies, its agility for change, and potential cultural barriers. An organization's culture can greatly influence the success or failure of new technology adoption.[1,2] Assessing cultural aspects is key before embarking on healthcare AI initiatives. This involves evaluating the organization's general willingness to adopt new technologies and processes. Some cultures eagerly embrace innovations, while others are more risk-averse. Understanding general attitudes toward change will inform the degree of culture shift needed.

Conducting an organizational readiness assessment in this manner highlights priority areas to address to smooth the path for implementing AI. The findings should guide an AI strategic roadmap aligned with the organization's strengths and needs.

Building an AI development team

Successfully building an AI development team in healthcare requires bringing together complementary skills and fostering collaboration.[3] The team should include both clinical and technical experts who can translate medical knowledge into robust AI models. Recruit healthcare professionals with expertise in the specific clinical area that AI is addressing to obtain vital insights into workflows and end-user requirements. Additionally, hire technically skilled AI modelers and developers to create the algorithms, data infrastructure, and applications. Project management skills can help coordinate across domains and maintain timelines. Fostering strong working relationships among team members is also important, as open communication and trust are essential when collaborating across disciplines. Particular attention should also be paid to the ethical composition of the team. Diversity in gender, race, socioeconomic status, and professional backgrounds will provide a wider range of viewpoints and considerations when designing healthcare AI. Overall, a cross-functional AI team with complementary abilities and a collaborative culture is the key to success.

Integration of AI models into clinical workflows

Implementing AI will inevitably disrupt established workflows and affect how clinicians spend their time.[4] Protocols should be developed collaboratively with clinicians to outline appropriate processes for AI-assisted decision-making, such as when to trust model recommendations versus seeking a second opinion. Change management strategies will be critical for adoption, such as extensive training on using new AI tools, clear communication about impacts on clinician time, and gathering regular feedback to improve integration. Leadership should assess clinician perceptions of the value AI adds to their workflows and monitor for burnout. With a human-centered approach that puts the needs of clinicians first, AI models can be integrated into practice more seamlessly. However, the process will require patience, iterative improvements, and a commitment to clinician engagement.

Monitoring, evaluating, and iterating on AI models

Ongoing monitoring, evaluation, and improvement are crucial to implementing AI models in healthcare. Rigorous frameworks should be created to continuously collect fresh data and assess real-world model performance through metrics like accuracy, precision, and model discrimination. This evaluation allows for the identification of model degradation and concept drift, which is when the predictive relationships the model was trained on change over time. To manage degradation, model retraining and calibration techniques must be applied through established iterative processes. Clinical teams should be engaged in regular model performance reviews and provide key insights on where further improvements are needed from a practice perspective. With comprehensive monitoring and established processes for keeping models up-to-date, the safety and effectiveness of AI systems can be maintained long after initial implementation. AI models in healthcare require ongoing vigilance and care to sustain their value.

Assessing ethical and legal issues in implementation

Additionally, the ethical and legal considerations surrounding patient data privacy and security must be carefully addressed to maintain patient trust and comply with regulations.[5,6] When implementing clinical AI systems, healthcare organizations must carefully address the ethical and legal considerations surrounding patient data privacy and security to maintain patient trust and comply with regulations. Conducting privacy impact assessments can identify potential data risks and document how patient information will be obtained, stored, accessed, and used throughout the AI model lifecycle. It is critical to review data regulations like HIPAA and GDPR to ensure collection and handling processes adhere to requirements around de-identification, encryption, consent, data minimization, and limitations on secondary data uses. A cybersecurity plan should outline steps to safeguard patient data through access controls, network security, encryption, and employee training. Principles of data minimization should be adopted by limiting the use of patient data to only what is essential for the AI model and restricting access to necessary personnel. Anonymizing or de-identifying patient data can further reduce privacy risks, as can techniques like differential privacy that preserves anonymity during AI model training. Transparency with patients about data usage and clear consent options are important, including allowing patients to opt out if desired. Processes for the continual auditing of data practices and AI systems can verify ongoing compliance with ethics policies and regulations. Establishing oversight bodies like patient data security boards and ethics advisory boards also provides governance and accountability around ethical data use. With concerted efforts to prioritize ethical data stewardship, healthcare organizations can implement clinical AI while upholding patient trust.

Assuring AI Safety

AI-enabled decision support systems, when implemented correctly, can aid in enhancing patient safety by improving error detection, patient risk stratification, and drug management. In a recent study by Eriksen *et al.*, for example, the authors used AI GPT-4 to diagnose complex medical cases.[23] The AI outperformed 99.98% of human readers. However, it is essential to verify these benefits.[7-9] While these controlled studies demonstrate the potential for AI to be highly accurate in healthcare settings, the real-world impact of implementing AI in clinical practice can only be determined after they are implemented into a healthcare system. The benefits of AI must be verified through real-world testing and evaluation after implementation.[10] Those implementing AI systems in healthcare bear the responsibility of ensuring patient health and safety are protected. This requires thoughtful integration into clinical workflows, extensive testing during development, monitoring performance post-deployment, and maintaining human oversight of AI-assisted decision-making.[11,12] Careful implementation and ongoing evaluation of clinical AI are crucial to realizing positive outcomes from these technologies.

System interoperability and integration

Interoperability and integration with existing healthcare systems are also critical considerations. AI applications need to seamlessly integrate with electronic health records (EHRs), clinical decision support systems, and other existing healthcare technologies.[13,14] Ensuring smooth data flow, standardization, and interoperability between different systems and platforms is crucial for the effective utilization of AI in clinical workflows.

Interoperability and integration can be achieved through the adoption of health information exchange standards and interoperability frameworks. Compliance with standards such as HL7 FHIR (Fast Healthcare

Interoperability Resources) facilitates seamless data exchange between different healthcare systems and promotes the integration of AI applications into existing clinical workflows.[15,16] Collaborating with IT departments and leveraging healthcare IT expertise can facilitate the successful integration of AI technologies into healthcare systems.

Economics

Demonstrating a positive economic impact is a critical factor when making the business case for or against investing in an AI solution in healthcare. The financial benefits of implementing an AI system, such as potential cost savings or revenue increases, must be compelling to justify the required investments in technology, training, and workflow integration. The potential for cost savings is a major motivation for adopting AI applications in healthcare. One estimate suggests that AI could reduce annual US healthcare expenditures by $150 billion by 2026.[17] A significant portion of these savings may come from shifting to a more preventative healthcare model enabled by AI, moving away from a purely reactive approach focused only on treatment. By facilitating proactive health management, AI applications could help decrease hospitalizations, doctor visits, and medical procedures through prevention and early intervention. This transition to a preventative system is expected to lower overall healthcare costs.

A rigorous analysis of the expected economic value versus implementation costs is essential for healthcare organizations to evaluate if the adoption of an AI solution makes strategic and financial sense. The economic impact projected by an AI vendor may not always match the actual impact once deployed, so healthcare leaders need to thoroughly assess both short-term costs and longer-term economic returns when deciding on AI investments.[17]

Addressing data quality and reliability

One significant challenge is ensuring the quality and reliability of data. AI models heavily rely on high-quality data to generate accurate predictions

and insights.[18] Before the data can be evaluated by the AI system, healthcare professionals must address data quality issues, such as missing data,
inconsistent formatting, and data biases, to ensure the reliability of AI
algorithms.[19] Regular data audits, data cleaning processes, and quality
assurance protocols can help ensure the reliability of data used for AI
algorithms. According to the 2022 American Health Information
Management Association's Health Care Data Governance practice brief,[20]
healthcare-related data used in AI systems should have the following
characteristics:

- Accuracy: The data should be free of errors and be correct.
- Accessibility: Proper safeguards are established to ensure data is
  available when needed.
- Comprehensiveness: The data contains all the required elements.
- Consistency: The data is reliable and the same across the entire patient
  encounter.
- Currency: Data is current and up to date.
- Definition: All data elements are clearly defined.
- Granularity: The data is at the appropriate level of detail.
- Precision: The data is precise and collected in its exact form.
- Relevancy: Data is relevant to the purpose it was collected.
- Timeliness: Documentation is entered promptly, is up to date, and
  available within the specified and required time frames.

Collaborations with data scientists and experts in data management
can assist healthcare professionals in developing effective data governance frameworks.

Practical guidance for healthcare professionals

To successfully incorporate AI into their workflow, healthcare professionals need to take several important steps.

First, they should have a clear understanding of the specific clinical
improvements or augmentations they want to achieve using AI. For
example, a physician specializing in radiology may want to improve the

accuracy of interpreting medical images using AI algorithms or an oncologist may collaborate with data scientists to develop an AI model that predicts patient response to different cancer treatments based on genetic data. Collaborating with AI experts and data scientists is key in this process. These professionals can provide valuable insights into selecting the appropriate AI models, developing customized algorithms, and tailoring them to specific clinical needs.

Healthcare professionals should also familiarize themselves with AI terminology and concepts to effectively communicate and collaborate with AI specialists. By understanding the fundamentals of AI, physicians can actively participate in discussions related to AI implementation and provide valuable input based on their clinical expertise. A cardiologist, for example, can collaborate with AI experts to discuss the importance of "feature selection" or "model evaluation metrics" when developing an AI model for predicting cardiovascular events.

Healthcare professionals need to be aware of the limitations and potential biases associated with AI algorithms.[21] While AI can provide valuable insights, it is not infallible. AI systems have "missed" lesions in imaging studies and have come to the wrong diagnosis after reviewing the patient's EMR. Physicians should critically evaluate AI-generated recommendations and be mindful of potential biases in the training data that may affect the algorithm's performance. For instance, a primary care physician using an AI-powered clinical decision support system should be aware of any biases in the data used to develop the system and carefully consider the recommendations in light of their knowledge and patient-specific factors.

Continuous education and training programs play a crucial role in empowering healthcare professionals to effectively incorporate AI into their clinical practice.[22] These programs can provide physicians with the necessary knowledge and skills to understand and evaluate AI technologies, interpret AI-generated results, and make informed decisions in collaboration with AI systems. For example, workshops or online courses can be offered to healthcare professionals to enhance their AI literacy and provide practical guidance on integrating AI technologies into their workflow.

By taking these steps, healthcare professionals can embrace AI technologies and leverage their potential to improve clinical decision-making, enhance patient outcomes, and drive advancements in healthcare. Collaborative efforts between healthcare professionals and AI experts are key to harnessing the power of AI effectively and responsibly in the clinical setting.

Strategies for successful integration and adoption

To ensure the successful integration and adoption of AI technologies in healthcare, healthcare professionals should follow a well-defined implementation strategy. Engaging stakeholders, including clinicians, administrators, and IT personnel from the early stages of planning is critical to fostering a comprehensive and collaborative approach. Clear communication channels should be established to facilitate effective collaboration and information exchange between different stakeholders. Regular feedback loops should be implemented to gather insights from end-users, such as physicians, regarding the ease of implementation, usability, and impact of AI technologies in their clinical practice. This feedback helps identify areas for improvement and allows for timely adjustments to optimize workflows and address any challenges that arise.

Pilot projects and phased implementation approaches are valuable strategies to assess the feasibility and impact of AI technologies before full-scale deployment. By conducting small-scale trials in specific clinical areas or departments, healthcare professionals can evaluate the performance and benefits of AI systems in real-world settings. As an example, a pilot project could involve testing an AI-powered diagnostic tool in a radiology department to assess its accuracy and efficiency in assisting radiologists with interpreting medical imaging scans. During the pilot phase, healthcare professionals can gather feedback from physicians regarding the usability, integration, and impact of the AI technology. This feedback informs adjustments and fine-tuning of the system based on the specific needs and preferences of the physicians and their clinical workflows.

Evaluating the effectiveness, usability, and impact of AI systems is essential to measure their value and guide further improvements. Robust evaluation frameworks and metrics should be established to assess the performance and outcomes of AI technologies. By way of illustration, physicians can provide feedback on the accuracy of AI-generated treatment recommendations or the impact of AI-driven decision support on patient outcomes. By collecting quantitative and qualitative data, healthcare professionals can assess factors such as diagnostic accuracy, treatment effectiveness, time-saving benefits, and overall user satisfaction. This evaluation process helps identify areas of success and areas that require further refinement or customization.

Overall, a well-defined implementation strategy, including stakeholder engagement, clear communication, pilot projects, and robust evaluation frameworks, ensures that AI technologies are successfully integrated into clinical practice. By involving physicians throughout the process and incorporating their feedback, healthcare professionals can tailor AI systems to meet the specific needs of physicians and enhance their ability to provide optimal patient care.

Conclusion

The integration of AI into healthcare holds great promise but also poses significant challenges that require thoughtful solutions. By taking a holistic approach that carefully assesses organizational readiness, assembles cross-disciplinary teams, centers clinical needs, and data quality, and prioritizes ethical data practices, healthcare institutions can implement AI successfully and responsibly. However, technological integration alone is not enough. The human components of change management, continuous improvement, and clinician engagement are equally critical. AI should augment, not replace, human intelligence and care in healthcare. With patient well-being at the core and humans firmly in control of technology, AI can become a collaborative partner in driving better health outcomes. By employing our humanistic strengths of wisdom, empathy, and ethics, the benefits of AI can be unlocked while minimizing its risks. Though the way forward is complex, it is a journey well worth undertaking together.

References

1. Prakash N. (2021) The influence of organizational culture on the adoption and diffusion of new technologies within firms. *Journal of Cardiovascular Disease Research*, **12**(6), 2190–2198.
2. Jackson S. (2011) Organizational culture and information systems adoption: a three-perspective approach. *Information and Organization*, **21**(2), 57–83.
3. Chen IY, Szolovits P, Ghassemi M. (2019) Can AI help reduce disparities in general medical and mental health care? *AMA Journal of Ethics*, **21**, 167–179.
4. Sendak D, Arcy J, Kashyap S, Gao M, Corey K, Ratliff B, Balu S. (2020) A path for translation of machine learning products into healthcare delivery. *Innovations — European Medical Journal*, doi: 10.33590/emjinnov/19-00172
5. Zhang J, Zhang Zm. (2023) Ethics and governance of trustworthy medical artificial intelligence. *BMC Medical Informatics and Decision Making*, **23**, 7.
6. Asan O, Bayrak AE, Choudhury A. (2020) Artificial intelligence and human trust in healthcare: focus on clinicians. *Journal of Medical Internet Research*, **22**(6), e15154.
7. Choudhury A, Asan O. (2020) Role of artificial intelligence in patient safety outcomes: systematic literature review. *JMIR Medical Informatics*, **8**(7), e18599.
8. Fernandes M, Vieira SM, Leite F, Palos C, Finkelstein S, Sousa JMC. (2020) Clinical decision support systems for triage in the emergency department using intelligent systems: a review. *Artificial Intelligence in Medicine*, **102**, 101762.
9. Yin J, Ngiam KY, Teo HH. (2021) Role of artificial intelligence applications in real-life clinical practice: systematic review. *Journal of Medical Internet Research*, **23**(4), e25759.
10. Maddox TM, Rumsfeld JS, Payne PRO. (2019) Questions for artificial intelligence in health care. *JAMA Network*, **321**(1), 31–32.
11. He J, Baxter SL, Xu J, Xu J, Zhou X, Zhang K. (2019) The practical implementation of artificial intelligence technologies in medicine. *Nature Medicine*, **25**(1), 30–36.
12. Juluru K, Shih HH, Keshava Murthy KN, Elnajjar P, El-Rowmeim A, Roth C, Genereaux B, Fox J, Siegel E, Rubin DL. (2021) Integrating AI algorithms into the clinical workflow. *Radiology: Artificial Intelligence*, **3**(6), e210013.

13. Davenport TH, Hongsermeier TM, Mc Cord KA. (2018) Using AI to improve electronic health records. https://hbr.org/2018/12/using-ai-to-improve-electronic-health-records
14. Alldus Recruitment. (2021) Electronic Health Records (EHRs): how AI is improving clinician use. https://alldus.com/blog/electronic-health-records-ehrs-how-ai-is-improving-clinician-use/
15. The complete guide to HL7. https://www.interfaceware.com/hl7-message-structure#:~:text=HL7%20Messages%20are%20used%20to,require%20some%20effort%20to%20interpret
16. HL7 FHIR foundation: enabling health interoperability through FHIR. https://fhir.org/
17. Wolff J, Pauling J, Keck A, Baumbach J. (2020) The economic impact of artificial intelligence in health care: systematic review. *Journal of Medical Internet Research*, **22**(2), e16866.
18. Refinitiv. (2019) Smarter humans. Smarter machines. Insights from the Refinitiv 2019 Artificial Intelligence/Machine Learning Global Study. https://www.refinitiv.com/content/dam/marketing/en_us/documents/gated/reports/refinitiv-ai-ml-survey-report.pdf#form
19. Ataman A. (2023) Data quality in AI: challenges, importance & best practices. https://research.aimultiple.com/data-quality-ai/
20. AHIMA. (2022) Healthcare data governance. https://www.ahima.org/media/pmcb0fr5/healthcare-data-governance-practice-brief-final.pdf
21. Gianfrancesco MA, Tamang S, Yazdany J, Schmajuk G. (2018) Potential biases in machine learning algorithms using electronic health record data. *JAMA Internal Medicine*, **178**(11), 1544–1547.
22. Garvey KV, Thomas Craig KJ, Russell R, Novak LL, Moore D, Miller BM. (2022) Considering clinician competencies for the implementation of artificial intelligence-based tools in health care: findings from a scoping review. *JMIR Medical Informatics*, **10**(11), e37478.
23. Eriksen AV, Möller S, Ryg J. (2023) Use of GPT-4 to diagnose complex clinical cases. *NEJM AI*, **1**(1), AIp2300031.

Chapter 13

Evaluating AI Models and Algorithms in Healthcare

The significance of evaluating AI models and algorithms in healthcare

In the ever-changing healthcare landscape, the integration of artificial intelligence (AI) holds great promise for improving patient outcomes and enhancing clinical decision-making. The primary goal of healthcare professionals is to provide the best care possible to their patients. Recognizing the importance of evaluating AI models and algorithms is key to unlocking the full potential of AI technology in healthcare settings and achieving that primary goal. Although the average clinician will not be performing these evaluations, it is important to understand them to increase trust in the systems, engage in collaboration with AI specialists, and make informed decisions about the reliability of the algorithm. This chapter aims to underscore the critical role of assessing the performance and reliability of AI models, emphasizing their profound impact on patient outcomes and clinical decision-making.

The power of accurate and reliable AI algorithms

Imagine having an AI assistant capable of navigating the vast sea of medical knowledge, providing accurate and reliable insights right at your fingertips. Such AI algorithms, when rigorously evaluated for performance, can be invaluable in accurately diagnosing diseases, predicting treatment responses, and assisting in complex decision-making processes. Like a skilled assistant, these accurate and reliable AI algorithms have the potential to revolutionize clinical practice, leading to improved patient outcomes.

Assessing performance of AI algorithms

To evaluate the performance of AI models, it is essential to understand key evaluation metrics. These metrics serve as the yardstick for measuring the accuracy and effectiveness of AI algorithms. One way of assessing the performance of an AI algorithm is by using a confusion matrix (Figure 1).

The confusion matrix is structured as a grid with four cells, representing four possible outcomes that provide a comprehensive view of the model's predictions and their corresponding actual outcomes (Figure 1). The contents of the four cells include:

- True Positives (TP): This cell indicates the number of instances where the model correctly predicted a positive outcome when the actual outcome was positive. In medical terms, this would correspond to correctly identifying a patient with a certain condition or disease.
- True Negatives (TN): This cell represents the number of instances where the model correctly predicted a negative outcome when the actual outcome was negative. In a medical context, this could refer to correctly identifying a healthy individual or ruling-out a particular diagnosis. One without the condition or disease under study.

	Actual Positive (P)	Actual Negative (N)
Predicted Positive (P′)	True Positive (TP)	False Positive (FP)
Predicted Negative (N′)	False Negative (FN)	True Negative (TN)

Figure 1.   Confusion Matrix

- False Positives (FP): This cell indicates the number of instances where the model incorrectly predicted a positive outcome when the actual outcome was negative. These are often referred to as "Type I errors." In medicine, this could correspond to a false diagnosis or a false positive test result.
- False Negatives (FN): This cell represents the number of instances where the model incorrectly predicted a negative outcome when the actual outcome was positive. These are often referred to as "Type II errors." In a medical context, this could mean failing to identify a patient with a condition or disease, leading to a missed diagnosis.

By examining the values in each cell of the confusion matrix, healthcare professionals can assess the performance of an AI model in terms of its ability to correctly classify and predict outcomes. Metrics, such as sensitivity, specificity, accuracy, precision and area under the receiver operating characteristic curve (AUROC), can be derived from the confusion matrix to further evaluate the model's performance and guide decision-making in healthcare settings. Think of these metrics as vital signs for assessing the performance of AI algorithms. They provide insights into the algorithm's ability to correctly identify true positives, true negatives, false positives, and false negatives — much like how vital signs help gauge a patient's health status.

Validation techniques: cross-validation and external validation

Validating AI models is essential to ensure their generalizability and reliability in healthcare. Just as seeking multiple medical opinions enhances diagnostic accuracy, employing validation techniques enhances the robustness of AI models. The two crucial validation techniques include cross-validation and external validation.

Cross validation, sometimes called K-Fold Cross Validation, involves dividing the available data into several subsets or "folds." Take for example, a dataset that is divided into five folds. The AI model is trained on four of the folds and tested on the fifth. This process is repeated five times, each time using a different fold as the test set. By analyzing the model's performance across all folds, the model's consistency and reliability can be evaluated (Figure 2). The AI model is trained on the training set and then evaluated on the corresponding test set.

This process is repeated multiple times, with each fold having a chance to act as a test set. By doing so, we simulate the model's performance on unseen data, just as a patient benefits from multiple doctors' insights. In the context of AI model evaluation, "unseen data" refers to data that the model has not been exposed to during the training phase.

Cross-validation helps us assess how well the AI model performs on different subsets of data and how it avoids overfitting. Overfitting is an undesirable machine learning behavior where the model becomes overly specialized to the training data and performs poorly on new data.

External validation, like seeking a second opinion from an independent expert, involves testing the AI model on a separate dataset. This dataset should be distinct from the one used for training and cross-validation. By doing so, the AI model is assessed on how well it performs in real-world scenarios, just like validating a medical opinion against an expert outside the initial consultation. External validation helps confirm the generalizability of the AI model and ensures that it performs well on new, unseen data. Consider an example where an AI model is developed to predict the risk of developing a certain medical condition based on genetic and lifestyle factors. After training the model on a large dataset and performing cross-validation, it is essential to conduct external validation using a separate dataset from a different population or healthcare institution. This external validation verifies the model's performance across diverse patient populations and increases its reliability and trustworthiness.

By employing cross-validation and external validation techniques, healthcare professionals can establish the generalizability and reliability of AI models. Similar to seeking multiple medical opinions, these techniques enhance diagnostic accuracy, validating AI models through these techniques strengthens their performance and ensures they can be applied effectively in real-world healthcare settings.

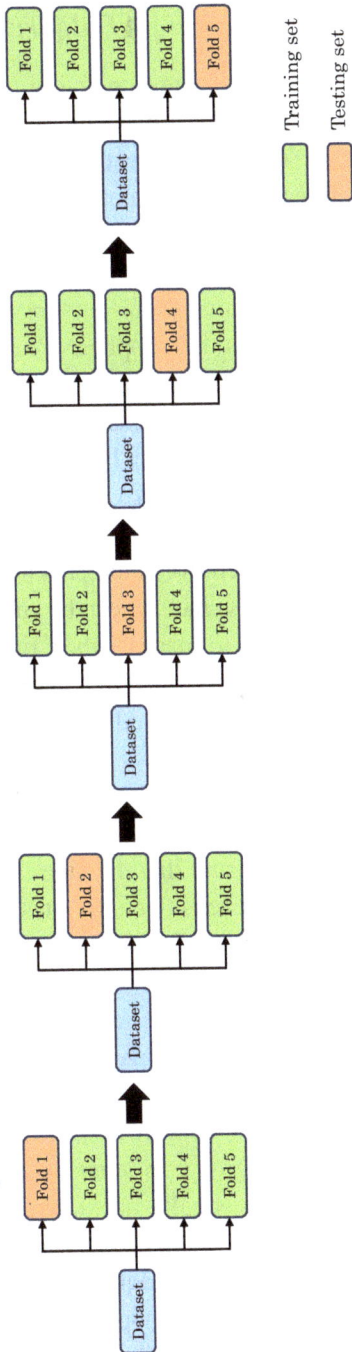

Figure 2. The data set is represented by the five tiles or folds. In each iteration of the cross-validation process, one fold (orange) is compared to the remaining folds (green). On the next cross validation, a different fold of data is compared to the remaining folds. This process is continued until each of the five folds has been compared to the rest.

Ethical considerations in evaluating AI algorithms

Healthcare professionals have an ethical responsibility to ensure fairness and mitigate biases in the AI algorithms that they employ. Just as healthcare professionals strive to provide equitable care to all their patients, it is imperative that the AI algorithms they use do not perpetuate biases or discriminate against certain populations.[1] Unfortunately, this does not always happen in AI models. Radiology studies have shown that AI imaging models can encode and learn patient-sensitive characteristics such as age, gender, and race.[2] When these models are applied to sub-groups (e.g., cross-validation), there can be significant disparities in performance.[3] Another example of bias is seen in the associations between the Framingham risk factors and cardiovascular events. Research has shown that risk factors can be significantly different across different ethnic groups.[4] Using the Framingham risk factors in all patient groups can lead to inaccurate risk stratification and inappropriate treatment for some patient groups.

To correct these disparities, fairness metrics can be employed. Fairness metrics are a way for an organization to measure their risk of exposure to machine learning bias and and their compliance to AI regulations. Fairness metrics are a group of common principles, guidelines, and standards that model developers adhere to.[5] Fairness metrics, such as equalized odds or predictive parity, can help assess and address potential biases in AI algorithms, aligning with a commitment to fairness and justice in patient care. These fairness metrics aim to ensure that the algorithm's predictions are not unfairly influenced by certain sensitive attributes, such as gender, race, or age.

- Equalized odds: Equalized Odds is a measure of fairness in machine learning, it evaluates whether the algorithm exhibits similar predictive performance across different groups defined by a sensitive attribute.[6] It examines whether the algorithm achieves equal rates of true positives and true negatives for each group. In other words, the algorithm should make predictions that are equally accurate for different sub-groups, irrespective of their sensitive attributes (e.g., race, gender, age, and medical condition). Achieving equalized odds helps avoid discriminatory practices where certain groups experience higher rates of false positives or false negatives.

- Predictive parity: Predictive parity focuses on the balance of positive outcomes predicted by the algorithm across different groups.[7] It aims to ensure that the algorithm's predictions do not disproportionately favor, or disadvantage specific groups based on sensitive attributes. The goal is to achieve a similar proportion of positive predictions (e.g., predicting the presence of a disease) for each group under consideration, regardless of their sensitive attributes. By maintaining predictive parity, the algorithm avoids creating or perpetuating disparities in healthcare outcomes among different population segments.

Regulatory and legal considerations in AI algorithms for healthcare

The evaluation and deployment of AI algorithms in healthcare are subject to various regulatory and legal considerations.[8] These guidelines and regulations play a crucial role in ensuring patient safety, data protection, and ethical use of AI technologies. Understanding the regulatory landscape is essential for healthcare professionals to navigate the complex environment of AI implementation in healthcare settings.

The regulatory landscape surrounding AI algorithms in healthcare is continually evolving. Regulatory bodies, such as the U.S. Food and Drug Administration (FDA), have recognized the need for specific frameworks to assess the safety, effectiveness, and reliability of AI algorithms in medical devices. For instance, the FDA has introduced a comprehensive framework to guide the development and evaluation of AI algorithms in medical devices, called the "Artificial Intelligence/Machine Learning (AI/ML)-Based Software as a Medical Device (SaMD) Action Plan" to promote transparency, accountability, and patient safety.[9]

The FDA's framework for AI in medical devices outlines key considerations for developers and healthcare professionals. It emphasizes the importance of defining the intended use and identifying the patient population for which the AI algorithm is intended. This framework requires manufacturers to establish a robust validation process, including collecting and evaluating real-world clinical data to demonstrate the algorithm's performance and safety.

Compliance with data protection and privacy regulations is another critical aspect when evaluating AI algorithms in healthcare. Healthcare organizations must adhere to regulations, such as the Health Insurance Portability and Accountability Act (HIPAA) in the U.S. or the General Data Protection Regulation (GDPR) in the European Union. These regulations ensure the protection of patient data, safeguarding privacy, and confidentiality. To comply with data protection and privacy regulations, healthcare professionals must carefully consider data governance, consent processes, and data anonymization techniques. It is vital to establish secure data storage and transmission practices to prevent unauthorized access or data breaches. Additionally, healthcare professionals must inform patients about the use of AI algorithms and ensure that appropriate consent is obtained.

Best practices for evaluating AI models and algorithms in healthcare

Evaluating AI models and algorithms in healthcare is a critical process that requires careful attention to ensure accuracy, validity, reliability, and ethical use. The evaluation of AI models and algorithms in healthcare requires a rigorous and systematic approach to ensure they are accurate, valid, reliable, and ethically applied.

To comprehensively evaluate an AI model's accuracy for healthcare use, its performance must be tested on datasets that closely represent real-world clinical data. The model should be run on multiple test sets that reflect the diversity of institutions and patient populations where it would be deployed. Metrics including sensitivity, specificity, AUROC, and predictive values should be calculated on each test set to quantify the model's ability to correctly detect the condition or outcome of interest. High accuracy on the original test data alone is not sufficient to ensure real-world viability.

Evaluating validity is a critical complement to accuracy testing. Validity assesses the model's ability to maintain accuracy on new test datasets that differ from the original training data. It tests the model's capability to generalize to varied data rather than memorizing patterns from the training data. Validity can be examined by evaluating model performance on test sets that have different distributions, demographics, patient numbers, and care settings compared to the training data. Significant declines in accuracy on new test data indicate potential biases and lack of validity. Comprehensive validity testing exposes these limitations and determines if the model is robust enough for broad clinical applications rather than narrow use cases.

Reliability refers to the consistency and reproducibility of an AI model's predictions over multiple runs, conditions, and time. A reliable model should produce very similar outputs given the same inputs. Lack of reliability indicates instability. Model instability refers to situations where an AI model produces inconsistent or highly variable outputs, predictions, or performance metrics across different conditions.

The ethical use of AI in healthcare also requires evaluating potential biases and harms. For example, are certain patient groups disproportionately misclassified? Does the model rely on proxies or attributes that could lead to discrimination? Broad and inclusive data, auditing for biases, and stakeholder consultation can uncover ethical risks. An extensive ethical evaluation through both technical and social/ethical lenses highlights the model's potential for direct or indirect harm before deployment. Employing these techniques demonstrates a commitment to "doing no harm" with AI in healthcare. Auditing and monitoring for ethical issues must continue post-deployment.

Healthcare professionals play a vital role in conducting robust evaluations to assess the performance and effectiveness of AI technologies. This section outlines the best practices for evaluating AI models and algorithms in healthcare, emphasizing transparency, reproducibility, and collaboration.

Transparency is a fundamental principle in evaluating AI models and algorithms. Healthcare professionals should strive to provide clear documentation of the AI model's development process, including data sources, preprocessing steps, and feature selection methods. Transparency allows for better understanding, scrutiny, and reproducibility of the results. An example of transparency is a scientific study where researchers provide detailed methodology and results, enabling other scientists to validate and build upon their findings. Similarly, transparent AI evaluations enable independent validation and promote the advancement of the field.

Reproducibility is another key aspect of robust evaluation. Reproducibility in AI means that an algorithm can be run repeatedly on certain datasets and obtain the same, or very similar, results each time. Healthcare professionals should ensure that their evaluation methods and code are well-documented and made publicly available whenever possible to encourage others to assess a model's reproducibility. By sharing code, datasets, and evaluation protocols, other researchers can replicate the evaluation process and verify the results. This fosters collaboration, allows for benchmarking against existing methods, and encourages the development of more reliable AI models. Reproducibility serves as the cornerstone of scientific progress, enabling the validation and improvement of AI algorithms.

Rigorous statistical methods are essential for accurate evaluation. Healthcare professionals should employ appropriate statistical techniques to analyze and interpret the performance metrics of AI models. This includes calculating metrics, such as accuracy, precision, recall, and F1 score, which provide insights into the model's performance across different evaluation scenarios. The F1 score is a metric used to evaluate the performance of binary classification models. A binary classification model is a type of machine learning model that is trained to make predictions on data with only two possible class labels or outcomes, such as, "Does the patient have the disease or not?" The F1 score is particularly useful when dealing with imbalanced datasets or situations where false positives and false negatives have different costs or implications (Figure 1). The F1 score is derived from two other metrics: precision and recall. Precision measures the proportion of true positive examples among all the examples that the model classified as positive, while recall measures the proportion of true positive examples among all the actual positive cases. The F1 score combines these two metrics to provide a balanced assessment of the model's ability to correctly classify positive and negative instances (Figure 1).

This type of statistical analysis ensures that evaluation results are robust, reliable, and free from bias.

Collaboration between healthcare professionals, data scientists, and regulatory bodies is essential for establishing evaluation standards and guidelines. These stakeholders should work together to define common evaluation protocols, performance metrics, and reporting guidelines. Collaboration allows for a comprehensive assessment of AI models and algorithms, considering diverse perspectives and expertise. By bringing together domain knowledge, technical expertise, and regulatory insights, collaboration ensures that the evaluations align with clinical needs, safety requirements, and ethical considerations.

Conclusion

In conclusion, evaluating AI models and algorithms in healthcare requires adherence to best practices. Transparency, reproducibility, and rigorous statistical methods are vital for conducting robust evaluations. Collaboration between healthcare professionals, data scientists, and regulatory bodies fosters the development of evaluation standards and guidelines that promote the reliable and ethical use of AI technologies. By following these best practices, healthcare professionals can confidently evaluate AI models and algorithms, paving the way for improved patient care and outcomes in the era of AI-driven healthcare.

References

1. Hooker S. (2021) Moving beyond "algorithmic bias is a data problem". *Patterns*, **2**(4), 100241.
2. Gichoya JW, Banerjee I, Bhimireddy AR, *et al.* (2022) AI recognition of patient race in medical imaging: a modeling study. *Lancet Digit Health*, **4**, e406–e414.
3. Seyyed-Kalantari L, Zhang H, McDermott MB, Chen IY, Ghassemi M. (2021) Underdiagnosis bias of artificial intelligence algorithms applied to chest radiographs in under-served patient populations. *Nature Medicine*, **27**, 2176–2182.
4. Gijsberts CM, Groenewegen KA, Hoefer IE, *et al.* (2015) Race/ethnic differences in the associations of the Framingham risk factors with carotid IMT and cardiovascular events. *PLoS One*, **10**(7), e0132321.
5. Mbakwe A, Lourentzou I, Celi LA, Wu JT. (2023) Fairness metrics for health AI: we have a long way to go. *EBioMedicine*, **90**, 104525.

6. Zhong Z. (2018) A tutorial on fairness in machine learning. https://towardsdatascience.com/a-tutorial-on-fairness-in-machine-learning-3ff8ba1040cb

7. Castelnovo A, Crupi R, Greco G, Regoli D, Penco IG, Cosentini AC. (2022) A clarification of the nuances in the fairness metrics landscape. *Scientific Reports*, **12**(1), 4209.

8. Gerke S, Minssen T, Cohen G. (2020) Chapter 12 — Ethical and legal challenges of artificial intelligence-driven healthcare. In *Artificial Intelligence in Healthcare*, Bohr A, Memarzadeh K (eds.), Academic Press, 295–336.

9. U.S. Food & Drug Administration. (2021) Artificial intelligence and machine learning in software as a medical device. https://www.fda.gov/medical-devices/software-medical-device-samd/artificial-intelligence-and-machine-learning-software-medical-device

Chapter 14

Human-Machine Interaction and User Experience Design in AI Systems for Healthcare

Introduction

Human-Machine Interaction (HMI) in the context of artificial intelligence (AI) systems refers to the collaboration and communication between the user and AI algorithms.[1] It involves the interaction, interface, and decision-making processes between humans and AI systems to improve medical decision-making and patient care. Imagine working with a knowledgeable assistant in a medical setting. This assistant is an AI system that can analyze oceans of patient data, provide insights, and assist in making accurate diagnoses and treatment recommendations. Similarly, the goal of HMI is to establish an effective partnership between healthcare professionals and AI systems, leveraging the strengths of both.

In this collaboration, healthcare professionals retain the final decision-making authority. While working alongside the AI system, they can consider its recommendations and insights, but should also be well aware of its limitation. The clinician can then independently evaluate and incorporate their expertise and judgment before making a decision. The AI system, therefore, serves as a valuable tool, augmenting the capabilities of healthcare professionals and enhancing the quality and efficiency of medical care.

The interaction between humans and AI systems in healthcare has many aspects, including interface design, communication channels, and the integration of AI insights into clinical workflows. It is very important to ensure that the AI system provides clear and interpretable results, communicates effectively with healthcare professionals, and aligns with their specific needs and requirements. By facilitating effective HMI, healthcare professionals can harness the power of AI to improve medical decision-making, enhance patient outcomes, and optimize the overall healthcare experience. The successful implementation of HMI in healthcare AI requires careful consideration of human factors, user experience design, and the unique context of medical practice. It is a collaborative and iterative process aimed at creating a harmonious partnership between humans and intelligent machines, ultimately benefiting both healthcare professionals and patients.

Before discussing User Experience Design (UXD), it may be helpful to define a "user interface." A user interface refers to the space or system through which interactions between humans and machines occur. It serves as a means for users to operate and control machines while receiving feedback and information simultaneously. The user interface encompasses interactive elements and components that enable users to interact with software applications, websites, operating systems, and various electronic devices. To illustrate the concept of a user interface, consider the following examples. Graphical user interfaces (GUIs) are commonly encountered in everyday use of smart phones, tablets, and computers. They utilize visual elements such as icons, buttons, and menus to facilitate user interaction. Command line interfaces (CLIs) rely on text-based commands for user input and feedback. Other examples include menu-driven interfaces, touch interfaces found in smartphones and tablets, and voice interfaces that respond to spoken commands. UXD is the process that design teams use to create products that provide meaningful and relevant experiences to users. It focuses on creating intuitive and user-friendly interfaces to enhance the overall experience of healthcare professionals when using AI systems.

In the context of healthcare, UXD plays a vital role in designing interfaces that are easy to use, efficient, and seamless for healthcare professionals.

The goal of UXD is to understand the needs, preferences, and workflows of healthcare professionals and translate that understanding into the design of interfaces that facilitate effective interactions with AI technology. This involves considering the specific challenges and requirements of physicians in their clinical practice and tailoring the design to meet those needs. By employing UXD principles, healthcare professionals can benefit from interfaces that are intuitive and user-friendly, allowing them to easily navigate and interact with AI systems. UXD aims to optimize the overall experience of healthcare professionals, making their interactions with AI technology more seamless and efficient.

Importance of user-centered design in AI systems for healthcare professionals

User-centered design is of paramount importance in the development and deployment of AI systems in healthcare.[2] Clinical decision support tools have often failed to improve patient outcomes because they are not well-integrated into clinical workflows, causing trigger alert fatigue or other unintended consequences.[3,4] By prioritizing the needs, preferences, and expertise of healthcare professionals, the user-centered design ensures that AI technology becomes a valuable tool rather than a source of frustration or confusion. User-centered design principles promote usability, efficiency, and satisfaction, leading to increased adoption and acceptance of AI systems among healthcare professionals. Additionally, involving healthcare professionals in the design process enhances system usability and accuracy, leading to better clinical outcomes. The user-centered design principles for AI systems in healthcare include:

Enhancing the healthcare worker's experience

In the rapidly evolving field of healthcare, the design of AI systems plays a crucial role in supporting physicians and optimizing patient care. This section explores user-centered design principles for AI systems in healthcare, focusing on the needs of healthcare professionals. By understanding and addressing these principles, AI systems can be tailored to enhance the experience of users, thereby leading to improved healthcare outcomes.

Understanding user needs and requirements in healthcare settings

To create effective AI systems, it is essential to thoroughly understand the needs and requirements of the users in healthcare settings. This involves engaging in user research and conducting in-depth interviews and observations to gain insights into the challenges that workers face. One possible challenge might include quick access to patient information and medical history when making critical decisions. Therefore, AI systems can be designed to provide timely and relevant information, so as to aid physicians in delivering accurate and efficient care.

Designing user-friendly interfaces for healthcare professionals

Well-designed user interfaces are essential for ensuring that healthcare workers can efficiently use and interact with AI systems. A user-friendly interface should present information in a clear and intuitive manner, minimizing cognitive load and enabling efficient decision-making. For instance, the user interface could organize patient data in a visually appealing and structured format, allowing physicians to quickly identify relevant information such as lab results, vital signs, and medication history. By prioritizing simplicity and ease of use, AI systems can enhance the workflow of physicians and reduce the likelihood of errors.

Incorporating clinician feedback and iterative design processes

Continuous feedback from clinicians is invaluable in refining and improving AI systems. By involving clinicians throughout the design and development process, their expertise can be leveraged to address usability issues and optimize system performance. Iterative design processes, such as usability testing and prototyping, allow clinicians to provide feedback on system functionality and suggest enhancements. This collaborative approach ensures that AI systems align with the specific needs of physicians, leading to greater acceptance and adoption. The alternate approach, where a user interface for a new AI system is foisted on healthcare professionals as a *fait accompli*, can result in confusion, resentment, and poor utilization of the system.

Balancing automation and user control in AI systems

An important consideration in AI system design is achieving the right balance between automation and user control.[5] While automation can streamline tasks and improve efficiency, it is essential to provide healthcare professionals with control over critical decisions. For instance, an AI system can suggest potential diagnoses based on patient symptoms and data, but the final diagnosis and treatment plan should remain in the hands of the healthcare professional. This balance ensures that clinicians maintain their expertise and judgment while benefiting from AI-driven insights.

Ensuring seamless integration of AI into clinical workflows

The successful integration of AI systems into existing clinical workflows is essential for their widespread adoption and effectiveness. AI should seamlessly fit into the established routines and processes of the clinicians, minimizing disruptions, and maximizing efficiency.[6,7] For example, AI systems can be integrated into electronic health record (EHR) systems, allowing physicians to access AI-generated recommendations within their familiar workflow. By seamlessly integrating AI, clinicians can leverage its potential while preserving the continuity of care.

Enhancing user experience in healthcare AI systems

As AI become more ubiquitous in healthcare settings, it is necessary to prioritize user experience (UX) in the design and implementation of these

AI systems. By considering visualizations and interaction paradigms for clinical decision support, designing intuitive interfaces for medical imaging, leveraging natural language processing and voice user interfaces for documentation and conversational AI, and personalizing AI tools for healthcare professionals, AI systems can be created to effectively support users and improve patient outcomes.

Visualizations and interaction paradigms for AI-driven clinical decision support

Data visualization involves creating graphical representations of information and data, such as charts, graphs, and maps. These data visualizations play a crucial role to aid healthcare professionals in comprehending complex AI-driven clinical decision-support outputs. Effective visual representations of data and insights enable healthcare professionals to interpret and make informed decisions based on AI-generated outputs.[8] Here are three key aspects to consider for enhancing the importance of visualizations:

Importance of visualizations

Visualizations serve as a bridge between raw data and meaningful insights, allowing healthcare professionals to grasp complex information quickly. By presenting data in a visual format, such as charts, graphs, or heatmaps, clinicians can identify patterns, trends, outliers, and anomalies at a glance. This visual understanding helps clinicians comprehend the underlying data and its implications, leading to more accurate diagnoses and treatment decisions. It was a data visualization that allowed Dr. John Snow to end a cholera epidemic in the So Ho district of London in 1854.[53] He marked the houses of the cholera victims on a street map. The map showed that the houses of the victims centered around a single water pump on Broad Street. He correctly concluded that the water from that pump must be the cause of the cholera outbreak and cut the handle off the pump, finally ending the epidemic.

Interactive interfaces

Intuitive and interactive interfaces enhance physicians' engagement with AI-generated insights and facilitate real-time exploration of data. These interfaces enable users to refine parameters, adjust algorithms, and explore different scenarios to better understand the impact of AI recommendations. By actively participating in the decision-making process, healthcare workers can leverage their expertise and judgment alongside AI-powered recommendations.

Contextualized visualizations

Contextual data visualization goes beyond just graphically depicting data to integrate relevant context. By presenting visual information within a meaningful framework, isolated data points can become connected into a comprehensible narrative.[9] This contextualization enables viewers to mentally relate disparate elements, fostering divergent analysis. The contextual relationships help reveal deeper insights into patterns, trends, and correlations that may be difficult to discern from the data alone. Effective contextual visualization not only presents data visually, but leverages context to render complex information more accessible, digestible, and actionable.

Consider a hypothetical example to illustrate this: Imagine being an environmental scientist who studies air quality in various cities across the globe. You collected raw data including levels of various pollutants like CO_2, NO_2, $PM2.5$, and others for each city over the past decade. Now, you wish to present your findings in a way that is easy to understand for policy-makers, environmental groups, and the public. A basic data visualization might be a set of line graphs for each city, plotting pollutant levels over time. While this may provide useful information, it is not particularly contextualized. In contrast, an interactive map could contextualize this data. The interactive map would display each city as a circle, where the size of the circle representing the overall pollution level. The color of the circle could indicate whether pollution is increasing or decreasing. Clicking on a city would open a detailed chart showing changes in each type of pollutant over time. Additionally, contextual information about significant events that might have influenced pollution levels could be included, such as the implementation of environmental regulations, industrial activities, or significant weather events. Moreover, data from other sources could be integrated for more context. For example, health data to show correlations between pollution levels and rates of respiratory illnesses in each city can be incorporated, or economic data could overlay to show the relationship between industrial activity and pollution. By integrating these various data sources into an interactive visualization, a more comprehensive and contextual view of the issue will be provided. This makes it easier for stakeholders to understand the full implications of the data that will aid them in making evidence-based decisions. Contextualized visualizations are tailored to specific clinical contexts, aligning with the needs and preferences of clinicians. By considering the unique requirements of different medical specialties, patient populations, and healthcare settings, visualizations can be designed to present relevant information in a manner that resonates with physicians' mental models. Contextualized visualizations enhance physicians' understanding and decision-making processes, as they can quickly identify and interpret information that is directly applicable to their specific clinical scenarios.

Designing intuitive and context-aware interfaces for AI-powered medical imaging

What is a context-aware interface?

Context-aware computing involves leveraging information about the user's situation and surroundings to dynamically adapt computer applications to better meet the user's needs.[10] By sensing contextual data such as a user's location, nearby devices, activity, relationships with other users, and operating environment, context-aware systems can provide more relevant, personalized experiences and services.[11] Context aware interfaces for healthcare AI systems are designed to integrate smoothly into clinical workflows and processes.[12] To do this effectively, they must understand existing healthcare workflows and be tailored to the specific needs, skills, and environments of the end users, whether physicians, nurses, or administrative staff. Rather than disrupt clinician workflows, context-aware AI interfaces adapt dynamically based on the clinical situation, user role, patient population, and other relevant contextual factors. This prevents alert fatigue and proactively surfaces the most relevant insights at the most appropriate time. Context-aware interfaces increasingly incorporate voice interactions and mobile accessibility to enable point-of-care use cases. The goal is to create intuitive, user-centered interactions that provide clinicians with helpful AI assistance without imposing additional cognitive burden or interrupting their work. By focusing on the clinical context and real workflow integrations, context-aware interfaces aim to drive adoption and utilization of healthcare AI.

A primary aspect of these interfaces is the ability to intelligently adapt their behavior based on the context of the situation. For example, such interfaces could consider the patient's medical history, the type of medical image being analyzed (e.g., MRI, CT, X-ray), the specific area of the body being imaged, and any known medical conditions relevant to the imaging. This context-awareness can enable the system to provide more accurate and personalized interpretations and predictions, hence facilitating better decision-making by clinicians.

Moreover, explainability and trustworthiness are important features of context-aware interfaces in medical imaging. Since there are high stakes in medical decisions, AI tools must provide recommendations that are transparent and can be understood by clinical stakeholders. The AI should not merely be a "black box" but rather provide clear reasoning for its conclusions, this fosters trust and allows for human oversight.

Context-aware interfaces can handle boundary-aware tasks, such as object detection, localization and edge detection.[13] These processes are involved in distinguishing and categorizing different parts of a medical image, which is crucial for clinical analysis and disease diagnosis. Boundary-aware context neural networks are designed to achieve more accurate segmentation masks and better understand the complex contextual relationships in medical images. These networks utilize advanced algorithms to identify and segment specific regions of interest within the image, aiding healthcare professionals in diagnosing conditions and planning treatments.

For instance, medical image segmentation can be instrumental in identifying and segmenting various organs, bones, or tumors from CT scans, MRIs, or other medical imaging modalities. By using context-aware interfaces and boundary-aware context neural networks, healthcare professionals can efficiently and precisely extract regions of interest from these images, facilitating accurate diagnosis and personalized treatment planning. Similarly, context-aware generative networks can perform tasks like estimating CT images from corresponding MR images.[14] By understanding the nonlinear relationship between MRI to CT, these networks can generate more realistic images.

Therefore, context-aware interfaces for AI-powered medical imaging are an important development in healthcare, which could significantly enhance the accuracy and utility of medical imaging technology. The critical advantage is their ability to incorporate relevant information about the context in which an image is analyzed, thereby providing more precise and personalized insights to support clinical decision-making. To harness the full potential of AI in medical imaging, it is crucial to design interfaces that are intuitive and context-aware.

Context-aware image analysis

AI interfaces must adapt to different imaging modalities, ranging from magnetic resonance imaging (MRI) to computed tomography (CT) and positron emission tomography (PET). Each modality offers unique information, from anatomical structures and morphology to physiological functions. Thus, the interface should seamlessly handle varying inputs and extract relevant insights. The interfaces should also adapt to diverse clinical scenarios. Algorithms could be designed to focus on certain aspects depending on the condition in question. For instance, AI can enhance sensitivity and specificity for detecting small radiographic abnormalities. A context-aware system is also crucial in addressing the type and biological aggressiveness of a lesion, which are aspects commonly overlooked in current AI imaging studies.

Workflow integration

The value of AI in medical imaging extends beyond diagnostic accuracy to include workflow efficiency.[15,16] Smooth integration of AI into existing radiology workflows is important in order to harness these benefits. An AI application should enhance automation in various imaging tasks without causing disruptions. As an example, consider the amount of patient data in the EHR that the average radiologist has to synthesize when planning the optimal image for a patient. This is where AI's ability to quickly scan and collate information into a meaningful plan based on the patient's clinical indication could be leveraged.[17] By optimizing the process of ordering studies, AI can reduce the number of unnecessary scans. In addition to optimizing imaging orders, AI could also assist with procedural details like patient positioning, contrast dosing, and scan sequencing. AI algorithms can incorporate patient factors like weight, kidney function, and mobility to provide personalized recommendations that improve safety and quality. By guiding appropriate contrast administration and positioning for each patient, AI can help reduce risks and errors. Over time, the improved safety and streamlining of imaging procedures enabled by AI guidance could also lower costs. Successful embedding of AI tools at different points throughout the radiology workflow in a simulated clinical environment has been demonstrated.[18] Such standards of interoperability should be incorporated in all future AI developments to ensure their seamless integration into current medical imaging workflows. Furthermore, radiologists should not need to exit their regular working window or log into a new system to use AI applications. A time-efficient, integrated workflow fosters physician satisfaction and enhances the acceptability of AI-powered decision support.

Real-time feedback

Real-time feedback is another critical aspect of an AI-powered medical imaging interface. Physicians should be able to validate AI-generated findings swiftly and, if necessary, correct them on the spot. This interaction between humans and AI can further improve the AI application by providing valuable learning experiences for the system.[19] Radiologists' feedback can be leveraged to fine-tune the AI-based image analysis algorithms and enhance the system's performance over time. Such a feature also ensures that the clinical insight and experience of healthcare professionals remain central to the diagnosis process, thus enhancing trust in AI systems.

Natural language processing and voice user interfaces for clinical documentation and conversational AI

Streamlining Clinical Documentation

Clinical documentation, while integral to patient safety, continuity of care, and quality improvement, can place a significant burden on healthcare professionals. The documentation involves routine work with written documents such as forms, records, or letters, and often detracts healthcare professionals from their primary role — delivering high-quality patient care.

The transition to EHRs in recent years has added complexity to the documentation process. As of 2015, 92% of hospital-based physicians were using EHRs. While EHRs have tremendous potential for improving healthcare delivery, their implementation has not been without challenges. One significant impact of EHRs is the increase in documentation burden, which, in turn, has been linked to the rise in burnout syndrome among clinicians. Documentation burden is often described as ill-defined and inconsistently measured, making it a significant challenge in the healthcare sector. It involves time-consuming data entry and administrative tasks that can significantly detract from patient care. In fact, physicians now spend up to twice as much time completing electronic documentation and administrative tasks (50%) as compared to time engaging in direct bedside patient care (12% to 27%).[20,21] Indeed, studies have shown that this "documentation burden" is associated with increased medical errors, documentation mistakes, patient safety concerns, job attrition, and emotional despair among health care providers.[22]

Natural language processing (NLP) may be one method to speed up documentation and counter provider burnout. NLP is an AI field that focuses on the conversion of unstructured human language data into structured data that machines can understand. By using NLP, clinical notes, patient interviews, and other types of unstructured data can be processed and understood by AI algorithms. This not only reduces the time physicians spend on administrative tasks but also enables more efficient care delivery by extracting actionable information from massive volumes of data. NLP methods can organize and evaluate the information contained in unstructured clinical notes, offering insights into patient care and the understanding of disease. In addition, clinical NLP systems can accurately model specific attributes and features, such as document content, adding another layer of analytical potential. A practical application of NLP is the development of a "contextual autocomplete" system,[23] which can aid physicians in their documentation by providing accurate and context-sensitive suggestions. This can significantly streamline the documentation process, reduce errors, and ultimately free up more time for direct patient interaction.

Conversational AI

Conversational AI encompasses the use of messaging apps, speech-based assistants, and chatbots to automate communication and deliver personalized customer experiences on a large scale.[24] This cutting-edge technology leverages AI and NLP to simulate human conversation. By analyzing the meaning of text and speech and generating contextually relevant responses, conversational AI systems can interact with users in a natural manner. The workings of conversational AI involve a combination of NLP and machine learning (ML). These AI systems are trained on very large amounts of data, including text and speech, which enable them to understand and process human language effectively. Continuously learning from user interactions, conversational AI improves its responses over time, ensuring an enhanced and personalized experience for customers.

In the healthcare sector, voice user interfaces are being employed to facilitate more natural and efficient interactions between physicians and AI systems.[25,26] These voice interfaces, often facilitated by AI, are not just limited to transcription services or command-and-response interactions.[27,28] They can understand context, consider the user's current situation, and offer a natural, conversational interaction. The primary objective here is to enable physicians to focus more on patient care rather than dealing with complex interfaces or searching through large amounts of data for necessary information.

For example, AI Voice Assistants in clinical documentation can help manage data entry work, freeing up clinicians to focus on medical decision-making and value-added care. AI Voice Assistants in clinical documentation refer to AI systems that help in the process of recording, transcribing, and analyzing healthcare encounters. They are a subset of intelligent conversational agents or virtual assistants, designed to aid healthcare service delivery, often used to increase efficiency and reduce the load of administrative tasks on healthcare providers.

These voice assistants can be utilized in various ways to improve clinical documentation. For instance, they can transcribe patient-provider conversations in real-time, analyze what is being said for medical relevance, cross-reference the conversation with the patient's holistic medical history and other available medical data, research, and best practices, and can even report findings and make diagnosis and treatment recommendations customized to the patient's situation. AI voice assistants can significantly reduce the amount of time physicians spend on administrative tasks, such as data entry, note creation, and reviewing medical records in EHR. This allows them to focus more on value-added care for their patients, promoting positive health outcomes and ensuring continuity of care.

Despite their benefits, these systems require careful management and ethical considerations. The patient's privacy must be secure and patients should have the option to opt out of being recorded at any time. It is also essential to ensure that medical decision-making remains primarily with clinicians, with AI acting as an assisting tool rather than the primary decision-maker.

Language understanding

Accurate interpretation of medical terminology and context-specific information is a critical requirement for AI systems used in healthcare. As much as 80% of all healthcare data is said to be unstructured, making it a challenge to interpret.[29,30] Unstructured data refers to information that does not adhere to a predefined data model or format. It contrasts with structured data, which is organized in a predictable, easily searchable manner, typically within databases. Unstructured data is characterized by its lack of organization in a fixed format, making it more challenging to collect, process, and analyze using conventional database technologies.

However, solving this issue would unlock an enormous amount of valuable information.

NLP systems can be instrumental in driving Clinical Decision Support (CDS), a process that aims to provide health-related information when it is needed. This could involve interpreting clinical narratives and presenting this information to physicians at the point of care, leading to better patient outcomes and more informed decision-making processes. To ensure accuracy, context is key. Therefore, systems need to consider contextual clues to comprehend words and phrases accurately.[31] For instance, a term like "MI" can mean myocardial infarction in one context and Michigan in another. Therefore, AI systems must be able to understand the context accurately in order to provide meaningful and valuable interpretations.

In summary, the integration of NLP and conversational AI in healthcare has the potential to revolutionize clinical documentation, enhance physician-patient interactions, and improve overall healthcare outcomes. The journey toward fully harnessing this potential is filled with exciting possibilities and transformative advances, which promises a future where technology significantly augments human capabilities in delivering care.

Personalization and customization of AI tools for individual healthcare professionals

Healthcare is experiencing a seismic shift driven by rapid advancements in technology and data analytics. This shift is profoundly transforming the sector, transitioning from a one-size-fits-all model to a personalized and customizable approach designed to fit individual preferences, needs, and outcomes. Within this context, AI emerges as a revolutionary tool capable of not only facilitating this change but also amplifying its benefits in healthcare.

Tailoring AI recommendations

AI systems hold significant potential for customization in healthcare, primarily through tailored recommendations. In practice, this approach implies that AI tools should adjust to individual physician preferences and clinical practice patterns, providing personalized suggestions. It allows clinicians to sift through enormous volumes of data and derive insights relevant to each patient's unique circumstances. With the help of machine learning algorithms, AI tools can create unique patient profiles and modify their recommendations accordingly. For example, patient management systems can prioritize information display based on a physician's preferred variables,[32] while diagnostic AI can tailor its prediction explanations to the physician's desired format, aiding in swift and accurate decision-making.

Adaptive learning

The field of adaptive learning, a facet of AI that evolves based on user interactions and individual feedback, is a boon to healthcare personalization.[33] Adaptive learning in the context of an AI system refers to the capability of the system to learn and evolve its behavior or responses based on new data or experiences. This concept is central to many AI applications, particularly in machine learning and deep learning. Adaptive learning in AI involves algorithms that adjust and improve over time, enhancing their performance and accuracy as they process more data. This dynamic functionality enables AI systems to continuously improve their recommendations based on individual feedback and outcomes. Through such adaptive learning processes, AI tools can refine their algorithms, grow more attuned to the healthcare professional's style, and deliver better patient care outcomes. The long-term goal is to create a positive feedback loop, wherein both the clinician and the AI tool learn from each other and improve over time.

User-driven customization

Incorporating user-driven customization into AI tools can foster a more personalized healthcare approach. Allowing healthcare professionals to customize AI interfaces and workflows empowers them to optimize AI system integration into their practice. Customizable AI interfaces make it possible for practitioners to align the AI system's operations with their unique practice workflows, eliminating unnecessary friction and enhancing overall productivity.[34] From simple interface elements like the arrangement of tools and features to more complex aspects like configuring AI-powered decision support systems, these customizable options ensure the AI serves as a seamless extension of the physician, rather than a disjointed and hard to use tool. Customization can be achieved based on data gathered from user preferences, browsing patterns, and interaction histories with the AI system.

E-health services have undergone significant enhancements through customization techniques, which have improved service delivery and accessibility. One prime example of e-health services adopting customization techniques is the National Health System (NHS) in the UK.[24] Through their online portal, they have been able to offer personalized services that have improved patient accessibility, increased efficiency, and enhanced patient engagement. Such advancements underscore the importance and effectiveness of personalization and customization in the field of healthcare.

Training healthcare professionals in using AI tools effectively

As the adoption and scaling up of AI in healthcare continue to increase, the need to adequately train health professionals in this emerging field becomes paramount. With aging populations, rising healthcare costs, and escalating demand for healthcare services, AI can augment the capacity of health professionals and improve the quality and delivery of healthcare services. This section explores various strategies for effectively training healthcare professionals in using AI tools.

Educational strategies for AI literacy and competency development

To successfully integrate AI into healthcare practices, health professionals need a solid understanding of AI technologies.[35,36] This involves fundamental education in AI technologies, ML, NLP, and AI voice assistants, among others. Introducing AI training in medical education and developing curricula to provide a foundational understanding of AI are essential. This includes not only the theoretical aspects of AI but also their practical implications and ethical considerations. Importantly, AI literacy should not be viewed as a specialized skill set, but rather a core competency for all healthcare professionals in the digital age.[37,38]

Hands-on training and simulation-based learning for AI applications

Beyond theoretical learning, health professionals need hands-on training and simulation-based learning to effectively use AI applications.[39] Practical exercises that emulate real-world scenarios can help learners to understand the potentials and limitations of AI, its interaction with human judgment, and its effects on patient outcomes. Furthermore, health professionals should be trained in interpreting AI outputs and integrating them into their clinical decision-making process. In addition, case-based training can help them understand the ethical and legal implications of using AI in patient care.

Addressing barriers and challenges in AI adoption and skill development

Several barriers and challenges hinder the widespread adoption of AI in healthcare and the development of AI-related skills among health professionals. These include a lack of skills, resistance to change, data privacy concerns, and potential digital inequity.[40,41] To address these barriers, it is essential to create an environment that encourages continuous learning and collaboration between different stakeholders.[42] Policymakers, educators, healthcare organizations, and AI developers should work together to develop strategies that facilitate the adoption of AI in healthcare.

Continuous professional development and lifelong learning in the AI era

The rapid evolution of AI technologies necessitates continuous professional development and lifelong learning among health professionals. AI in healthcare is a continually evolving field, and professionals need to stay updated on the latest developments. AI-focused continuing medical education programs, workshops, and seminars should be made accessible for practicing professionals. Additionally, fostering a culture of self-directed learning will empower health professionals to take charge of their learning journey in the AI era.

Human factors and usability evaluation in healthcare AI

Usability testing and evaluation of AI systems in clinical settings

The usability principle for medical AI tools emphasizes that clinicians and other end-users should be able to efficiently and safely apply such tools to achieve clinical goals in their actual work environments.[43] Usability testing in this context refers to the evaluation of how easily and effectively end-users can interact with and utilize these systems. This process is essential for ensuring that AI applications are user-friendly, intuitive, and meet the needs of their intended audience. As the application of AI within healthcare continues to grow, there is a growing need for usability testing and evaluation of these systems within clinical settings.[44,45] Ensuring effective and reliable interactions between humans and machine is imperative, particularly given the direct impact that these systems can have on patient outcomes. Usability testing involves both technical and user-centered evaluation approaches. Technical testing primarily focuses on ensuring the system functions as expected, while user-centered approaches involve assessing how easily healthcare professionals can interact with the AI system, interface design, understandability of the AI's outputs, and overall user experience. This is vital to ensure a smooth integration of the technology into healthcare practice. It also includes evaluating how well the system supports clinical workflow, its impact on productivity, and its influence on the quality of care provided.

Assessing user satisfaction, acceptance, and trust in AI tools

The widespread implementation of AI within healthcare is largely dependent on its acceptance by healthcare professionals.[46] This acceptance is influenced by a range of factors, including the perceived usefulness and ease of use of the AI system, its reliability, and the training and support available for users.[48] Trust is another important factor, with users needing to feel confident that the AI system can reliably support their decision-making processes.[49] Assessing user satisfaction involves collecting feedback from users about their experiences with the AI system. This can be done through interviews, surveys, or observational studies. Additionally, metrics such as system usage rates, error rates, and time spent interacting with the system can provide valuable insights into user acceptance and satisfaction.

User-centered evaluation metrics for AI performance and clinical outcomes

Evaluating the performance of AI systems in healthcare goes beyond simple technical measurements of accuracy or speed. It also includes assessing the impact of the system on clinical outcomes and user experience.[50] User-centered evaluation metrics may include factors like user satisfaction, user acceptance, system usability, and how the system influences clinical decision-making. In addition, more outcome-focused metrics can be used, such as changes in patient health status, improvements in care quality, reductions in clinical errors, or improvements in care efficiency.

Incorporating human factors engineering principles in AI system design

Human factors and ergonomics (HF/E) play a crucial role in the design and development of AI systems in healthcare.[51] These principles focus on understanding human psychological, social, physical, and biological characteristics and using this information to design systems that optimize human performance, health, and safety. Applying HF/E principles in the design of AI systems helps to ensure that the technology is user-friendly, supportive of clinical workflow, and designed with user needs and capabilities in mind.[52] This involves engaging healthcare professionals early in the design process to understand their needs, work processes, and the challenges they face. This user-centered design approach helps to ensure that the AI system is integrated smoothly into the clinical setting, thereby leading to improved acceptance, satisfaction, and trust in the technology.

As the use of AI in healthcare continues to expand, the need for rigorous human factors and usability evaluation becomes increasingly critical. These processes ensure that AI tools not only perform their intended functions but also integrate effectively into the clinical workflow, meet the needs of healthcare professionals, and ultimately improve patient outcomes.

Conclusion

The role of human-machine interaction and user experience design is central to the successful implementation of AI systems in healthcare. The convergence of human expertise and AI computational power can deliver superior outcomes, provided the interaction is effective in promoting collaboration rather than over-reliance. To achieve this, there is a need for thoughtful design and management of AI systems, considering both the technical and human aspects. These systems should be integrated seamlessly into clinical workflows, with a keen focus on optimizing user experience. Acknowledging the social aspects of human-AI interaction and including end-users in the design process are critical steps to ensure that the technology is useful, trustworthy, and accepted by healthcare professionals and patients alike. As AI continues to impact healthcare, robust research into ethical deployment and parameter setting for AI usage will further enhance the team-working approach between humans and machines. The future of healthcare AI hinges on this crucial interaction, highlighting the need for continuous improvement in user experience design and human-machine interaction.

References

1. Jabeen H. (2023) HMI technologies: the ultimate guide to human-machine interface innovations. https://www.wevolver.com/article/hmi-technologies-the-ultimate-guide-to-human-machine-interface-innovations

2. Gillies M, Fiebrink R, Tanaka A. (2016) Human-centred machine learning. *Proceedings of the 2016 CHI Conference Extended Abstracts on Human Factors in Computing Systems*, Association for Computing Machinery, New York, NY, USA, 3558–3565.

3. Stone EG. (2018) Unintended adverse consequences of a clinical decision support system: two cases. *Journal of the American Medical Informatics Association*, **25**, 564–567.

4. Cohen JP, Cao T, Viviano JD, *et al.* (2021) Problems in the deployment of machine-learned models in health care. *Canadian Medical Association Journal*, **193**, E1391–E1394.

5. Heer J. (2019) Agency plus automation: designing artificial intelligence into interactive systems. *Proceedings of the National Academy of Sciences of the United States of America*, **116**(6), 1844–1850.

6. Blezek DJ, Olson-Williams L, Missert A, Korfiatis P. (2021) AI integration in the clinical workflow. *Journal of Digital Imaging*, **34**(6), 1435–1446.

7. Juluru K, Shih HH, Keshava Murthy KN, Elnajjar P, El-Rowmeim A, Roth C, Genereaux B, Fox J, Siegel E, Rubin DL. (2021) Integrating AI algorithms into the clinical workflow. *Radiology: Artificial Intelligence*, **3**(6), e210013.

8. Levy-Fix G, *et al.* (2019) Machine learning and visualization in clinical decision support: current state and future directions. https://arxiv.org/pdf/1906.02664.pdf

9. Zheng RZ, Greenberg K. (2019) What is contextual visualization. In *Leveraging Computer Interface to Support Creative Thinking.* https://www.igi-global.com/dictionary/contextual-visualization/65827#:~:text=Contextual%20visualization%20refers%20to%20a,whole%20image%20through%20mental%20association

10. Zon M, Ganesh G, Deen MJ, Fang Q. (2023) Context-aware medical systems within healthcare environments: a systematic scoping review to identify subdomains and significant medical contexts. *International Journal of Environmental Research and Public Health*, **20**(14), 6399.

11. Abowd GD, Dey AK, Brown PJ, Davies N, Smith M, Steggles P. (1999) Towards a better understanding of context and context-awareness. In *Handheld and Ubiquitous Computing. HUC 1999. Lecture Notes in Computer Science, vol 1707*, Gellersen HW. (ed.), Springer, Berlin, Heidelberg, 304–307.

12. Bricon-Souf N, Newman CR. (2007) Context awareness in health care: a review. *International Journal of Medical Informatics*, **76**(1), 2–12.

13. Wang R, Chen S, Ji C, Fan J, Li Y. (2022) Boundary-aware context neural network for medical image segmentation. *Medical Image Analysis*, **78**, 102395.

14. Nie D, Trullo R, Lian J, Petitjean C, Ruan S, Wang Q, Shen D. (2017) Medical image synthesis with context-aware generative adversarial networks. *Medical Image Computing and Computer Assisted Intervention — MICCAI* 2019, **10435**, 417–425.

15. Benefits of artificial intelligence to radiology workflows. https://healthitanalytics.com/news/benefits-of-artificial-intelligence-to-radiology-workflows

16. Kapoor N, Lacson R, Khorasani R. (2020) Workflow applications of artificial intelligence in radiology and an overview of available tools. *Journal of the American College of Radiology*, **17**(11), 1363–1370.

17. Song J. (2021) Using artificial intelligence to improve radiology workflow. https://www.thedoctors.com/articles/using-artificial-intelligence-to-improve-radiology-workflow/

18. Dikici E, Bigelow M, Prevedello LM, White RD, Erdal BS. (2020) Integrating AI into radiology workflow: levels of research, production, and feedback maturity. *Journal of Medical Imaging (Bellingham)*, **7**(1), 016502.

19. Frąckiewicz M. (2023) The role of AI in medical imaging: a new vision for diagnosis. https://ts2.space/en/the-role-of-ai-in-medical-imaging-a-new-vision-for-diagnosis/

20. Poissant L, Pereira J, Tamblyn R, *et al.* (2005) The impact of electronic health records on time efficiency of physicians and nurses: a systematic review. *Journal of the American Medical Informatics Association*, **12**, 505–516.

21. Colicchio TK, Cimino JJ. (2019) Clinicians' reasoning as reflected in electronic clinical note-entry and reading/retrieval: a systematic review and qualitative synthesis. *Journal of the American Medical Informatics Association*, **26**, 172–184.

22. Moy AJ, Schwartz JM, Chen R, *et al.* (2021) Measurement of clinical documentation burden among physicians and nurses using electronic health records: a scoping review. *Journal of the American Medical Informatics Association*, **28**, 998–1008.

23. Gopinath D, Agrawal M, Murray L, *et al.* (2020) Fast, structured clinical documentation via contextual autocomplete. *Proceedings of Machine Learning Research*, **106**, 1–26.

24. Conversational AI: what is it and how does it work? https://www.247.ai/insights/conversational-ai-what-it-and-how-does-it-work

25. Singh B. (2023) The future of voice technologies in healthcare. https://www.forbes.com/sites/forbestechcouncil/2023/02/13/the-future-of-voice-technologies-in-healthcare/?sh=6a09385519ba

26. Jadczyk T, Wojakowski W, Tendera M, Henry TD, Egnaczyk G, Shreenivas S. (2021) Artificial Intelligence can improve patient management at the time of a pandemic: the role of voice technology. *Journal of Medical Internet Research*, **23**(5), e22959.

27. Kutty S. (2021) The rise of AI voice assistants in clinical documentation. https://www.forbes.com/sites/forbesbusinesscouncil/2021/03/03/the-rise-of-ai-voice-assistants-in-clinical-documentation/?sh=386c79e656cc

28. Dasgupta S. (2023) How integrating AI into clinical documentation can ensure precise coding compliance while maximizing reimbursement rates. https://www.linkedin.com/pulse/how-integrating-ai-clinical-documentation-can-ensure-precise-shaonli/

29. SyTrue. (2015) Why unstructured data holds the key to intelligent healthcare systems. https://hitconsultant.net/2015/03/31/tapping-unstructured-data-healthcares-biggest-hurdle-realized/

30. Pak HS. (2018) Unstructured data in healthcare. https://artificial-intelligence.healthcaretechoutlook.com/cxoinsights/unstructured-data-in-healthcare-nid-506.html.

31. Matson M. (2023) Semantic analysis: AI terms explained. https://www.playerzero.ai/advanced/ai-terms-explained/semantic-analysis-ai-terms-explained

32. Tajgardoon M, Cooper GF, King AJ, Clermont G, Hochheiser H, Hauskrecht M, Sittig DF, Visweswaran S. (2020) Modeling physician variability to prioritize relevant medical record information. *JAMIA Open*, **3**(4), 602–610.

33. Petersen C, *et al.* (2021) Recommendations for the safe, effective use of adaptive CDS in the US healthcare system: an AMIA position paper. *Journal of the American Medical Informatics Association*, **28**(4), 677–684.

34. Neuhauser L, Kreps G, *et al.* (2013) Using design science and artificial intelligence to improve health communication: ChronologyMD case example. *Patient Education and Counseling*, **92**(2), 211–217.

35. (2020) Why healthcare professionals need to understand AI. https://www.zmescience.com/medicine/healthcare-understand-ai-05223/#:~:text=The%20benefits%20of%20understanding%20AI&text=If%20doctors%20understand%20the%20abilities,a%20specific%20condition%2C%20for%20example

36. Lomis K, Jeffries P, Palatta A, Sage M, Sheikh J, Sheperis C, Whelan A. (2021) Artificial intelligence for health professions educators. *National Academy of Medicine Perspectives*, 2021:10.31478/202109a.
37. Kolachalama VB, Garg PS. (2018) Machine learning and medical education. *npj Digital Medicine*, **1**, 2–4.
38. Grunhut J, Marques O, Wyatt ATM. (2022) Needs, challenges, and applications of artificial intelligence in medical education curriculum. *JMIR Medical Education,* **8**, 1–5.
39. Dave M, Patel N. (2023) Artificial intelligence in healthcare and education. *British Dental Journal*, **234**(10), 761–764.
40. Ronen O. (2023) Obstacles to widespread adoption of AI in the healthcare industry. https://www.spiceworks.com/tech/innovation/guest-article/obstacles-of-ai-in-healthcare-industry/
41. Singh R, Hom G, *et al.* (2020) Current challenges and barriers to real-world artificial intelligence adoption for the healthcare system, provider, and the patient translational vision science & technology. *Translational Vision Science & Technology*, **9**(2), 45.
42. Arlinghaus T, Kus K, Behne A, Teuteberg F. (2022) How to overcome the barriers of AI adoption in healthcare: a multi-stakeholder analysis. *PACIS 2022 Proceedings*, 4, 1300. https://aisel.aisnet.org/pacis2022/4
43. Usability. (2023) https://future-ai.eu/principle/usability/
44. Park Y, Jackson GP, Foreman MA, *et al.* (2020) Evaluating artificial intelligence in medicine: phases of clinical research. *JAMIA Open*, **3**(3), 326–331.
45. Kushniruk AW, Patel VL. (2004) Cognitive and usability engineering methods for the evaluation of clinical information systems. *Journal of Biomedical Informatics*, **37**(1), 56–76.
46. Lambert SI, Madi M, Sopka S, *et al.* (2023) An integrative review on the acceptance of artificial intelligence among healthcare professionals in hospitals. *npj Digital Medicine*, **6**, 111.
47. Noyes J. (2023) Perceptions of AI in healthcare: what professionals and the public think. https://www.tebra.com/theintake/medical-deep-dives/tips-and-trends/research-perceptions-of-ai-in-healthcare
48. So S, *et al.* (2021) Exploring acceptance of artificial intelligence amongst healthcare personnel: a case in a private medical centre. *International Journal of Advances in Engineering and Management*, **3**(9), 56–65.
49. Asan O, Bayrak AE, Choudhury A. (2020) Artificial intelligence and human trust in healthcare: focus on clinicians. *Journal of Medical Internet Research*, **22**(6), e15154.

50. Reddy S, Rogers W, Makinen VP, Coiera E, Brown P, Wenzel M, Weicken E, Ansari S, Mathur P, Casey A, Kelly B. (2021) Evaluation framework to guide implementation of AI systems into healthcare settings. *BMJ Health & Care Informatics*, **28**(1), e100444.

51. Sujan M, *et al.* (2021) Human factors and ergonomics in healthcare AI. https://www.researchgate.net/publication/354728442_Human_Factors_and_ Ergonomics_in_Healthcare_AI?channel=doi&linkId=6149f540519a1a381f 75ce0d&showFulltext=true

52. Asan O, Choudhury A. (2021) Research trends in artificial intelligence applications in human factors health care: mapping review. *JMIR Human Factors*, **8**(2), e28236.

53. Tulchinsky TH. (2018) John Snow, Cholera, the Broad Street Pump; Waterborne Diseases Then and Now. In *Case Studies in Public Health*, 77–99.

54. NHS. https://www.nhs.uk/

Chapter 15

Patient Perspectives and Engagement with AI in Healthcare

Introduction

Artificial intelligence (AI) has emerged as a transformative technology with the potential to revolutionize healthcare. Its applications in diagnostics, treatment planning, and patient care hold tremendous promise for improving medical outcomes and enhancing the overall patient experience. However, successful implementation of AI in healthcare relies not only on technical advancements but also on understanding and addressing the perspectives of patients, who are at the center of the healthcare ecosystem.[1,2] Since patients stand to benefit from many AI innovations in healthcare, it is important to thoroughly understand patients' needs, values, and priorities. Doing so will help ensure that these advances are ethically developed and implemented in ways that improve patient care, rather than just being well-received. Widespread patient distrust of AI systems could result in result in implementation failure, and customer loss.[3]

This chapter aims to delve into the critical topic of patient perspectives and engagement with AI in healthcare. By exploring the attitudes, beliefs, concerns, and expectations of patients regarding the use of AI technologies, we can gain valuable insights that inform the development, deployment, and ethical considerations associated with AI in healthcare.

This chapter will also explore patients' perceptions of human-AI interaction, their attitudes toward clinical AI, and the factors that influence their acceptance of AI technologies.

Key themes that will be addressed in this chapter include patient apprehensions about AI, potential barriers to patient acceptance, patient understanding of AI technologies, privacy and security concerns, and the impact of AI on patient-provider relationships. Additionally, this chapter delves into the role of patient engagement in the development and evaluation of AI-driven healthcare solutions, emphasizing the importance of involving patients in decision-making processes and design considerations.

It is essential for healthcare professionals to be equipped with this knowledge as they navigate the evolving landscape of AI in healthcare and strive to deliver patient-centered care in an era of technological advancements.

Exploring patients' attitudes, perceptions, and expectations regarding AI technologies

Patients play a central role in healthcare, and their attitudes, perceptions, and expectations regarding AI technologies are crucial for the successful implementation and adoption of AI in healthcare settings.

Patients' beliefs, concerns, and acceptance of AI in healthcare

Several studies have examined patients' beliefs, concerns, and acceptance of AI technologies in healthcare. A 2019 survey found that most patients were open to AI technologies being used in their care but had concerns about data privacy and wanted to know how these systems work.[4] These studies have shed light on the perspectives of patients and the public towards AI, both in hypothetical scenarios and real-world implementations. The literature review conducted by Young and Amara in their 2021 Lancet article provides a comprehensive overview of patient and public attitudes towards clinical AI, including quantitative, qualitative, and mixed methods original research articles.[5] They found that patients and the public had a generally positive disposition towards AI technologies in healthcare. However, their acceptance of AI was tempered by concerns and apprehensions, as they valued the presence of human involvement and supervision in the context of AI-enabled healthcare interventions.

Patient apprehensions and potential barriers

Understanding patient apprehensions and potential barriers is essential for addressing concerns and promoting the acceptance of AI in healthcare. Studies have identified many of these apprehensions and potential barriers, including privacy concerns, lack of understanding, trust issues, and ethical implications.[6,7] Patients understand that the complexities of healthcare today require extensive sharing and access to their health information. This sharing exacerbates their privacy concerns because it expands the availability of patient data to numerous members of the healthcare team. These concerns may cause the patients to withhold important clinical information from their caregivers. The results of a national survey of patients published in American Medical Informatics Association's Annual Symposium Proceedings in 2020 revealed an inverse relationship between patients' trust in their provider and their willingness to withhold clinical information.[8] These apprehensions and barriers can impact patient engagement with AI technologies and hinder their acceptance.

Areas of interest related to AI implementation

Patients have expressed interest in specific areas where AI can enhance healthcare delivery. Indeed, AI-based applications that assist in disease detection, medical advice, clinical decision-making, and diagnostics have drawn particular attention. Patients recognize the potential of AI technologies to improve healthcare outcomes and streamline processes, which can lead to better patient care and experiences.[9]

Factors influencing patients' attitudes and expectations

Patients' attitudes and expectations towards AI technologies in healthcare are influenced by various factors.[10] These factors include digital affinity, sociodemographic characteristics, health-related factors, and psychosocial correlates. Understanding these factors is essential for healthcare professionals when tailoring AI implementations in a way that aligns with patients' needs and preferences.

Digital affinity

Digital affinity refers to the individuals' familiarity, comfort, and proficiency with digital technologies. Patients who are more technologically savvy and have positive experiences with digital tools may have a higher acceptance and positive attitude towards AI technologies in healthcare. Conversely, patients who are less familiar with or have negative experiences with technology may exhibit more skepticism or resistance.[11]

Sociodemographic characteristics

Sociodemographic factors such as age, gender, education level, and socioeconomic status can influence patients' attitudes and expectations toward AI in healthcare. For example, younger individuals who have grown up with technology may be more open to AI innovations, while older individuals may be more cautious or hesitant. Similarly, education level and socioeconomic status can impact patient's access to and understanding of AI technologies, which can, in turn, shape their attitudes.

Health-related factors

Patients' health conditions, experiences with healthcare, and perceived benefits of AI technologies can also influence their attitudes. For instance, patients with chronic illnesses who have struggled with complex treatment regimens may be more receptive to AI tools that can provide personalized support and guidance. Additionally, patients who have had positive experiences with previous AI applications in healthcare may have higher expectations and more favorable attitudes toward future implementations.

Psychosocial correlates

Psychosocial factors, including trust in technology, perceived control, privacy concerns, and ethical considerations, play a significant role in shaping patients' attitudes towards AI in healthcare. Trust in the accuracy, security, and reliability of AI algorithms and systems is crucial for patient acceptance. Privacy concerns regarding the collection and use of personal health data can also influence attitudes. Patients' sense of control over their healthcare decisions and the extent to which AI technologies are perceived as empowering or threatening can impact their expectations and attitudes. Examples include:

- A young, tech-savvy patient with a chronic illness may embrace AI technologies that offer personalized treatment recommendations and remote monitoring capabilities, viewing them as valuable tools to improve their health management.
- An older patient with limited technological experience and lower socioeconomic status may exhibit skepticism towards AI technologies due to unfamiliarity and concerns about accessibility or potential biases.
- A patient who has previously experienced privacy breaches in the healthcare system may express concerns about data security and be hesitant to adopt AI technologies that require sharing personal health information.
- A patient with a strong sense of autonomy and preference for human interaction in healthcare decision-making may resist AI technologies that they perceive as replacing the human touch.

By considering these factors and addressing patients' specific needs, healthcare professionals can ensure that AI implementations are patient-centered and effectively meet their expectations and preferences.

Involving patients in the development and evaluation of AI-driven healthcare solutions

Involving patients in the development and evaluation of AI-driven healthcare solutions is essential for creating patient-centered and effective technologies. Patient engagement ensures that the solutions address the specific needs and preferences of the individuals who will benefit from them. This section explores strategies, frameworks, and successful case studies that highlight the importance of patient involvement in AI research and implementation.

Exploring strategies and frameworks for patient engagement

To effectively engage patients in the design, development, and evaluation of AI-driven healthcare solutions, various strategies and frameworks have been proposed. These approaches provide guidance on how to involve patients throughout the entire process. For example, the systematic review by Bombard *et al.* in the journal Implementation Science,[12] identifies strategies and contextual factors that enable optimal engagement of patients in the design, delivery, and evaluation of health services. These strategies may include establishing patient advisory groups, involving patients in decision-making processes, and ensuring clear communication channels. Additionally, scoping reviews have explored models and frameworks of patient engagement in health services research, offering valuable insights into best practices. To illustrate, Chudyk *et al.* published a scoping review in the British Medical Journal examining models and frameworks guiding patient engagement in health services research.[13] These models provided structured approaches to involving patients at various stages of research, ensuring their perspectives are integrated into decision-making and evaluation processes.

Case Studies

Several case studies and projects have successfully incorporated patient involvement in AI research and implementation. These examples demonstrate the positive impact of patient engagement on the development of AI-driven healthcare solutions.

A successful case study that highlights patient involvement in AI research and implementation is the project conducted by Skovlund *et al.* in the journal Research Involvement and Engagement.[15] This study explored the impact of patient and public involvement (PPI) throughout the entire research process, including analysis. The collaboration between patients, researchers, and healthcare professionals had significant implications for research outcomes and the experiences of all stakeholders involved. The researchers employed a patient engagement approach in their primary care research, aiming to make the research more relevant and valuable to patients. The researchers worked in collaboration with the Canadian Institutes of Health Research's Strategy for Patient-Oriented Research and the Patient Engagement Resource Centre. By involving patients with lived experience of the disease and establishing a research advisory group, the study ensured that patients played a vital role in AI model-building and decision-making processes.

Through their involvement, patients provided valuable insights and perspectives, ensuring that AI technologies aligned with their needs, expectations, and values. The study demonstrated the benefits of patient involvement in implementation research, emphasizing the importance of incorporating patient perspectives to improve the adoption and acceptance of AI technologies in healthcare. By evaluating patient engagement, researchers and healthcare professionals can continuously improve the incorporation of patient perspectives in AI-driven healthcare solutions.

By actively engaging patients, healthcare professionals and researchers can ensure that AI technologies are user-friendly, effective, and aligned with patient preferences and values. Metaphorically, involving patients in the development and evaluation of AI-driven healthcare solutions is like building a bridge between technological advancements and human experiences. Patients' active participation provides the necessary support pillars, ensuring that the bridge is sturdy, functional, and capable of carrying the weight of their needs and expectations. By involving patients, the bridge becomes a collaborative effort, with patients providing valuable insights and guidance to create a seamless connection between AI technologies and personalized care.

Strategies for effective patient education and communication about AI in medicine

Patient education and communication play a vital role in fostering trust, understanding, and acceptance of AI technologies in healthcare.[16] Effectively conveying AI concepts, benefits, limitations, and potential risks to patients is essential for promoting informed decision-making and ensuring successful implementation. This section discusses the importance of patient education and communication in building a solid foundation of knowledge and trust regarding AI in medicine. Furthermore, it examines approaches and best practices for effective communication of AI concepts to patients.

Importance of patient education and communication

Patient education and communication play an important role in healthcare, empowering patients to take an active role in their care and promoting patient-centered approaches. Effective patient education goes beyond providing instructions and information, but also involves assessing patient needs, concerns, readiness to learn, preferences, and support systems. By fostering clear and meaningful communication, healthcare providers and educators can ensure that patients are equipped with the knowledge and understanding necessary to make informed decisions about their health and participate in their treatment plans.

- Fostering trust and understanding: Patient education and communication are key to building trust between healthcare providers and patients.[17] Transparent and clear communication about AI technologies helps patients understand the role of AI in their care, dispelling misconceptions and establishing realistic expectations. When patients are well-informed, they can actively engage in shared decision-making and feel empowered in their healthcare journey.
- Enhancing informed decision-making: Educating patients about AI concepts, benefits, limitations, and potential risks enables them to make informed decisions regarding their treatment options.[18] By providing accurate and accessible information, healthcare providers can

support patients in understanding how AI technologies can complement traditional approaches, improve diagnosis and treatment, and enhance overall healthcare outcomes.

Approaches and best practices for effective communication

Effective communication is a vital skill that plays a fundamental role in various aspects of life, including personal relationships, professional interactions, and teamwork. By employing appropriate strategies and best practices for communication, individuals can enhance their ability to connect, collaborate, and convey their messages more effectively. Developing effective communication skills involves being clear, attentive, empathetic, and understanding to foster meaningful and productive interactions.

- Use plain language: Using simple and jargon-free language is imperative when communicating with patients about AI. Research has shown that most doctors use language that is too complex for patients to understand,[19] highlighting the need for clear and concise explanations. By employing plain language, healthcare providers can bridge the knowledge gap and ensure patients comprehend AI concepts and their implications.
- Visual aids and infographics: Incorporating visual aids and infographics can enhance patient understanding of AI concepts and processes. Visual representations help simplify complex ideas, making them more accessible and memorable. Infographics can effectively convey information about AI benefits, risks, and potential outcomes. By presenting information visually, healthcare providers can engage patients and facilitate comprehension.
- Tailor information to individual patients: Recognizing that patients have diverse backgrounds, health literacy levels, and information preferences is essential. Healthcare providers should adapt their communication style and content to meet the specific needs of each patient. By understanding patients' perspectives and tailoring the information accordingly, providers can ensure that patients grasp AI concepts and feel more comfortable with its implementation in their care.

- Highlight ethical considerations: Given the ethical implications of AI in medicine, it is important to discuss these considerations with patients. Transparency about data privacy, algorithmic bias, and the importance of human oversight in decision-making can address potential concerns and enhance patient trust. Openly addressing ethical aspects fosters a collaborative environment where patients feel valued and involved in shaping AI-driven healthcare solutions.
- Continuous engagement and feedback: Patient education about AI in medicine should not be a one-time occurrence. Healthcare providers should establish channels for ongoing communication and feedback to address patients' questions, concerns, and evolving information needs. Regular updates, educational materials, and opportunities for dialogue enable patients to stay informed and actively participate in the integration of AI technologies into their care.

Ethical considerations and privacy concerns in patient engagement with AI

Ethical considerations and privacy concerns associated with patient engagement in AI-driven healthcare are of paramount importance. To ensure the responsible and ethical implementation of AI in healthcare, it is necessary to address these concerns. Guidelines and frameworks play a key role in establishing practices that prioritize privacy, informed consent, and data protection in AI research and implementation. By examining existing guidelines and frameworks, healthcare organizations can develop robust strategies to address these considerations and promote ethical practices in patient engagement with AI-driven healthcare.

One primary area of concern revolves around the access, use, and control of patient data in the context of AI-driven healthcare. With many AI technologies being owned and controlled by private entities, the implementation of AI can raise privacy issues and data security challenges. Protecting patient privacy and ensuring data security should be a top priority when leveraging AI in healthcare settings. Obtaining informed consent is another important concern and it is central in AI-driven healthcare. Patients should have a clear understanding of how their data will be used, the potential implications, and the benefits they can expect from AI applications in their healthcare journey. Guidelines and frameworks can provide recommendations for obtaining informed consent that aligns with ethical principles and legal requirements. Additionally, data protection is a critical aspect of AI research and implementation in healthcare. It is essential to implement measures that safeguard patient data, prevent unauthorized access, and ensure secure data storage and transmission. Guidelines and frameworks can offer insights into best practices for data protection in the context of AI-driven healthcare.

By addressing ethical considerations and privacy concerns and following established guidelines and frameworks, healthcare organizations can navigate the complex landscape of AI-driven healthcare while upholding patient rights, privacy, and data protection. These efforts contribute to building trust, promoting responsible AI adoption, and ensuring the ethical use of AI in patient engagement.

Evaluating the impact of patient engagement on AI-driven healthcare

Patient engagement has emerged as a pivotal factor in the implementation and success of AI-driven healthcare. Evaluating the impact of patient engagement on AI-driven healthcare outcomes, such as patient satisfaction, treatment adherence, and health outcomes, provides valuable insights into the effectiveness of involving patients in their healthcare journey. Several studies have assessed the influence of patient engagement on healthcare quality and identified positive outcomes associated with patient involvement in AI-driven healthcare.[20]

A scoping review in the September 2022 Journal of Patient Experience[21] on the topic of patient engagement and healthcare quality revealed that patient engagement strategies implemented by pharmaceutical and medical device companies have the potential to affect treatment decisions, care outcomes, and overall healthcare quality. According to a Bombard study in Implementation Science, engaging patients in the design, delivery, and evaluation of health services is recognized as an essential approach to improving health outcomes, enhancing patient satisfaction, and reducing costs.[12] Moreover, active patient participation and empowerment contribute to reduced healthcare expenses, optimal resource utilization, and improved patient-provider satisfaction. Patient engagement initiatives have demonstrated positive effects on AI implementation in healthcare.

However, patients have many concerns, too.[22] These include concerns related to the safety of AI, threats to patient choice, increases in healthcare costs occasioned by increased technology costs, bias in the datasets, and privacy of patient data. While patient concerns about the use of AI in healthcare exist, addressing these concerns through patient engagement is crucial for successful implementation. Engaging patients in discussions and decision-making regarding the use of AI technologies can alleviate apprehensions and improve acceptance. Moreover, patient engagement plays a significant role in increasing medication adherence, a critical aspect of treatment success and health outcomes. By involving patients in their care and leveraging AI technologies, healthcare providers can support patients in adhering to prescribed treatment regimens, leading to improved health outcomes.

Successful examples of patient engagement initiatives in AI-driven healthcare exist across various domains. For instance, the use of mobile device applications tailored to specific healthcare pathways has shown positive outcomes in patient engagement, satisfaction, and reported outcomes in a study sponsored by Apple.[23] Patients were provided with a mobile app that guided them through preoperative preparation, in hospital recovery, and post-op discharge care with personal reminders and task lists and education showing high engagement and satisfaction scores following robotic surgery in a study published in the Journal of Thoracic Disease.[24] In another study, mobile app-based interventions to support diabetes self-management resulted in clinically significant reductions in HbA_{1c}.[25] These initiatives provide personalized guidance, reminders, educational resources, and progress tracking, empowering patients to actively participate in their recovery process. Such initiatives contribute to enhanced patient engagement and improved healthcare experiences. Reviewing studies that assess the impact of patient engagement on AI-driven healthcare outcomes reveals positive associations with patient satisfaction, treatment adherence, and health outcomes. Successful patient engagement initiatives demonstrate the benefits of involving patients in decision-making, promoting adherence, and improving healthcare quality. By prioritizing patient engagement, healthcare providers can maximize the potential of AI in delivering personalized and patient-centered care.

Future directions and recommendations

As the field of AI continues to advance, there are several areas for further research and improvement in patient engagement with AI technologies. Additionally, there is a need for recommendations to enhance patient perspectives and involvement in AI-driven healthcare solutions. This section provides insights into these future directions and offers recommendations for healthcare providers, researchers, and policymakers.

Research directions

- Evaluation of patient experience: Further research is needed to assess the impact of AI technologies on patient experience and satisfaction. This includes studying the usability, acceptability, and perceived benefits of AI-driven healthcare solutions from the patient's perspective. Understanding patient experiences will help identify areas for improvement and inform the development of patient-centered AI tools.
- Ethical and legal considerations: There is a need to address ethical and legal considerations related to AI technologies in healthcare. Research should focus on understanding the privacy and security concerns associated with patient data, ensuring transparency and accountability in AI algorithms, and addressing potential biases or discrimination in AI-driven decision-making processes.
- Long-term outcomes and safety: Studies should investigate the long-term outcomes and safety of AI-driven interventions. This includes evaluating the effectiveness, reliability, and potential risks or adverse events associated with AI technologies. Longitudinal studies can provide valuable insights into the impact of AI on patient outcomes and guide the development of evidence-based practices.

Recommendations

- Patient-centered design: Healthcare providers, researchers, and developers should prioritize patient-centered design principles when creating AI-driven healthcare solutions. This includes involving patients in the design and development process, considering their needs, preferences, and values, and ensuring the usability and accessibility of AI technologies for diverse patient populations.

- Transparent and explainable AI: AI algorithms used in healthcare should be transparent and explainable to both patients and healthcare providers. Patients should have access to understandable explanations of AI-driven recommendations or decisions, empowering them to make informed choices and participate in shared decision-making processes.

- Informed consent and shared decision-making: Healthcare providers should ensure that patients are well-informed about the use of AI technologies in their care. This includes obtaining informed consent for AI-driven interventions, explaining the potential benefits and limitations, and involving patients in shared decision-making processes to jointly determine the best course of action.

- Education and empowerment: Patients should be provided with education and resources to enhance their understanding of AI technologies and their implications in healthcare. This includes promoting health literacy, facilitating patient access to trustworthy information about AI, and fostering patient empowerment in navigating and utilizing AI-driven healthcare solutions.

- Policy and regulation: Policymakers should establish guidelines and regulations to govern the development, deployment, and use of AI technologies in healthcare. These policies should address issues such as data privacy, security, algorithmic transparency, and patient rights. Collaboration between policymakers, healthcare providers, researchers, and patient advocacy groups is crucial to ensure that AI-driven healthcare solutions prioritize patient well-being and adhere to ethical standards.

The future of patient engagement with AI technologies in healthcare relies on ongoing research, patient-centered design, ethical considerations, transparency, informed consent, shared decision-making, patient education, and appropriate policies to enhance patient perspectives and involvement, ultimately maximizing the potential benefits of AI in improving healthcare outcomes.

Conclusion

In this chapter, the attitudes, perceptions, and expectations of patients regarding AI technologies in healthcare were explored. Through a review of various studies, we have gained valuable insights into patients' beliefs, concerns, and acceptance of AI in healthcare. It is evident that patient engagement is essential in the development and evaluation of AI-driven healthcare solutions. By involving patients in the design process, we can ensure that the technologies meet their needs and address their concerns.

Effective patient education and communication about AI in medicine have been identified as essential strategies. By providing clear and accessible information on AI concepts, benefits, limitations, and potential risks, we can enhance patient understanding and foster trust. Moreover, ethical considerations and privacy concerns must be addressed to ensure patient rights and data protection. Patient engagement in AI-driven healthcare has the potential to impact outcomes positively. Research has indicated that patient involvement can lead to increased satisfaction, improved treatment adherence, and better health outcomes. By considering patient perspectives and involving them in decision-making processes, we can create healthcare systems that prioritize patient-centered care.

References

1. Concannon TW, *et al.* (2014) A systematic review of stakeholder engagement in comparative effectiveness and patient-centered outcomes research. *Journal of General Internal Medicine*, **29**, 1692–1701.
2. Laï MC, Brian M, Mamzer M. (2020) Perceptions of artificial intelligence in healthcare: findings from a qualitative survey study among actors in France. *Journal of Translational Medicine*, **18**(1), 14.
3. Muthukrishnan N, *et al.* (2020) Brief history of artificial intelligence. *Neuroimaging Clinics of North America*, **30**, 393 (2020).

4. Nadarzynski T, Miles O, Cowie A, Ridge D. (2019) Acceptability of artificial intelligence (AI)-led chatbot services in healthcare: a mixed-methods study. *Digital Health*, **5**, 2055207619871808.

5. Young AT, Amara D, *et al.* (2021) Patient and general public attitudes towards clinical artificial intelligence: a mixed methods systematic review. *The Lancet Digital Health*, **3**, e599–e611.

6. Tyson A, Pasquinin G, Spenser A, *et al.* (2023) 60% of Americans would be uncomfortable with provider relying on ai in their own health care. https://www.pewresearch.org/science/2023/02/22/60-of-americans-would-be-uncomfortable-with-provider-relying-on-ai-in-their-own-health-care/

7. Richardson JP, Smith C, Curtis S, *et al.* (2021) Patient apprehensions about the use of artificial intelligence in healthcare. *npj Digital Medicine*, **4**, 140.

8. Iott BE, Campos-Castillo C, Anthony DL. (2020) Trust and privacy: how patient trust in providers is related to privacy behaviors and attitudes. *AMIA Annual Symposium Proceedings*, **2019**, 487–493.

9. Khullar D, Casalino LP, Qian Y, Lu Y, Krumholz HM, Aneja S. (2022) Perspectives of patients about artificial intelligence in health care. *JAMA Network*, **5**(5), e2210309.

10. Richardson JP, Curtis S, Smith C, Pacyna J, Zhu X, Barry B, Sharp RR. (2022) A framework for examining patient attitudes regarding applications of artificial intelligence in healthcare. *Digital Health*, **8**, 20552076221089084.

11. Chalutz Ben-Gal H. (2023) Artificial intelligence (AI) acceptance in primary care during the coronavirus pandemic: What is the role of patients' gender, age and health awareness? A two-phase pilot study. *Frontiers in Public Health*, **10**, 931225.

12. Bombard Y, Baker GR, Orlando E, *et al.* (2018) Engaging patients to improve quality of care: a systematic review. *Implementation Science*, **13**, 98.

13. Chudyk AM, Horrill T, Waldman C, Demczuk L, Shimmin C, Stoddard R, Hickes S, Schultz AS. (2022) Scoping review of models and frameworks of patient engagement in health services research. *BMJ Open*, **12**(8), e063507.

14. Vat LE, Finlay T, Robinson P, Barbareschi G, Boudes M, Diaz Ponce AM, Dinboeck M, Eichmann L, Ferrer E, Fruytier SE, Hey C, Broerse JEW, Schuitmaker-Warnaar TJ. (2021) Evaluation of patient engagement in medicine development: A multi-stakeholder framework with metrics. *Health Expect*, **24**(2), 491–506.

15. Skovlund PC, Nielsen BK, Thaysen HV, *et al.* (2020) The impact of patient involvement in research: a case study of the planning, conduct and

dissemination of a clinical, controlled trial. *Research Involvement and Engagement*, **6**, 43.

16. Al Kuwaiti A, Nazer K, Al-Reedy A, Al-Shehri S, Al-Muhanna A, Subbarayalu AV, Al Muhanna D, Al-Muhanna FA. (2023) A review of the role of artificial intelligence in healthcare. *Journal of Personalized Medicine*, **13**(6), 951.

17. Asan O, Yu Z, Crotty BH. (2021) How clinician-patient communication affects trust in health information sources: temporal trends from a national cross-sectional survey. *PLoS One*, **16**(2), e0247583.

18. Tran V-T, Riveros C, Ravaud P. (2019) Patients' views of wearable devices and AI in healthcare: Findings from the ComPaRe e-cohort. *npj Digital Medicine*, **2**, 53.

19. Gotlieb R, Praska C, Hendrickson MA, *et al.* (2022) Accuracy in Patient Understanding of Common Medical Phrases. *JAMA Network*, **5**(11), e2242972.

20. Wale JL, Chandler D, Collyar D, Hamerlijnck D, Saldana R, Pemberton-Whitely Z. (2022) Can we afford to exclude patients throughout health technology assessment? *Frontiers in Medical Technology*, **3**, 796344.

21. Marzban S, Najafi M, Agolli A, Ashrafi E. (2022) Impact of patient engagement on healthcare quality: a scoping review. *Journal of Patient Experience*, **9**, 23743735221125439.

22. Richardson JP, Smith C, Curtis S, *et al.* (2021) Patient apprehensions about the use of artificial intelligence in healthcare. *npj Digital Medicine*, **4**, 140.

23. jamf. (2018) Global research from Jamf reveals hospital mobile device initiatives increase patient satisfaction. https://www.jamf.com/resources/press-releases/global-research-from-jamf-reveals-hospital-mobile-device-initiatives-increase-patient-satisfaction/

24. Kneuertz PJ, Jagadesh N, Perkins A, Fitzgerald M, Moffatt-Bruce SD, Merritt RE, D'Souza DM. (2020) Improving patient engagement, adherence, and satisfaction in lung cancer surgery with implementation of a mobile device platform for patient reported outcomes. *Journal of Thoracic Disease*, **12**(11), 6883–6891.

25. Wu Y, Yao X, Vespasiani G, Nicolucci A, Dong Y, Kwong J, Li L, Sun X, Tian H, Li S. (2017) Mobile app-based interventions to support diabetes self-management: a systematic review of randomized controlled trials to identify functions associated with glycemic efficacy. *JMIR mHealth uHealth*, **5**(3), e35. Erratum in: *JMIR mHealth uHealth*, **6**(1), e20.

Chapter 16

AI and Clinical Decision Support

Definition and purpose of a clinical decision support system

A clinical decision support system (CDSS) is a health information technology that provides clinicians, staff, patients, and other individuals with knowledge and person-specific information to assist in making informed decisions regarding patient care at the point in time that these decisions are made.[1] It encompasses a variety of tools designed to enhance decision-making within the clinical workflow.[5] These tools aid clinicians in making informed decisions, promoting adherence to best practices, and reducing errors. To be clear, clinical decision support (CDS) algorithms are prediction models. These models are used to estimate the likelihood of potential patient outcomes or categorize patients' risk levels, rather than provide definitive "yes or no" answers. CDS algorithms make these calculations based on certain input variables like a patient's age, existing health conditions, and lab test results. Importantly, the predictions generated by CDS take the form of probabilities, not binary conclusions. They only determine, for example, if a diagnosis is more or less likely. However, many physicians erroneously treat these nuanced probabilistic predictions as if they are black-and-white answers. It is very important for doctors to recognize the inherent uncertainty in CDS predictions and to incorporate them appropriately into clinical decision-making. Rather than viewing a CDS-generated 30% risk of sepsis as a confirmed sepsis diagnosis, healthcare professionals should see it as a probability estimate that warrants further evaluation and testing. Avoiding the temptation to equate CDS predictions with definitive diagnoses will lead to better clinical decision-making and patient care. The nuanced, probabilistic nature of CDS output must be accounted for by clinicians seeking to make well-informed, evidence-based decisions.

The purpose of a CDSS is to improve the quality of patient care, enhance patient safety, and optimize clinical outcomes. It achieves these goals by integrating clinical knowledge, patient data, and evidence-based guidelines to provide timely and relevant information at the point of care. CDSS tools can include computerized alerts and reminders, clinical guidelines, condition specific order sets, patient data reports, documentation templates, diagnostic support, and contextually relevant reference information.[2] By leveraging artificial intelligence (AI) and machine learning techniques, CDSS can analyze large volumes of patient data, such as medical records, laboratory results, and imaging studies, to generate personalized recommendations and predictions. These systems can identify potential medication errors, alert clinicians about drug interactions or allergies, suggest appropriate diagnostic tests, and recommend treatment options based on best practices and patient-specific factors. Computerized CDSSs generate predictions that physicians then interpret and act on. How doctors respond to CDS predictions substantially affects patient care. For example, sepsis alert systems analyze real-time patient data to identify early signs of sepsis that most physicians would not have detected through clinical observation alone. When physicians respond quickly to CDS alerts regarding potential sepsis cases, the patient's likelihood of survival can increase significantly.[3] CDSS can improve decision-making by providing clinicians with valuable support and assistance in complex healthcare scenarios.[4] CDSS can reduce errors, prevent adverse events, and promote evidence-based practice.[5] They can help healthcare providers stay updated with the latest medical knowledge, guidelines, and research findings, ultimately leading to more informed and effective patient care. Additionally, CDSS can assist in standardizing care practices, improving workflow efficiency, and supporting the training of medical professionals.[6,7]

However, it is important to note that while CDSS can provide valuable support and recommendations, it should not replace a healthcare provider's clinical judgment and expertise. Clinicians should always exercise their professional judgment and consider individual patient characteristics and preferences when making decisions. CDSS should be seen as a tool to augment decision-making rather than replacing the role of a healthcare provider.

Overview of the development of CDSS

In 1959, the concept of using computers to aid in medical decision-making was first proposed. The authors of this idea speculated that computers could potentially execute intricate reasoning tasks, gather and process clinical data, and alert physicians to diagnoses that might have been missed.[67] Since its first use in the 1980s, CDSS has undergone significant development and evolution in healthcare. CDSS emerged as a groundbreaking technology that aimed to augment clinicians in their complex decision-making processes.[8] Over the years, CDSS adoption has been facilitated by the increasing global adoption of electronic medical records and computerized clinical workflows. These systems are designed to analyze electronic health records, integrate knowledge, and deliver patient-specific information to clinicians. The growth of CDSS has been driven by government initiatives, such as the US's Health Information Technology for Economic and Clinical Health (HITECH) Act of 2009, which incentivized the implementation of health information systems and CDSS.[9] To ensure that these systems were safe, effective, and unbiased, the Food and Drug Administration began regulating them.[10] Today, CDSS continues to evolve, with ongoing research and development aimed at enhancing their effectiveness, optimizing patient outcomes, and addressing potential risks and challenges.

As technology continues to advance, CDSS will likely further evolve and incorporate emerging AI technologies (e.g., wearable monitors, computer vision, and clinical prediction models). These advancements will expand the applications of CDSS in various domains of healthcare and beyond. The historical development of CDSS since the 1980s has transformed the healthcare landscape, empowering clinicians with sophisticated tools and knowledge to make more informed decisions, enhance patient outcomes, and improve the overall quality of care.

Components and functionality of Clinical Decision Support Systems (CDSS)

CDSS can be based on one of the two types of AI systems — knowledge-based AI and data-driven AI.

Knowledge-based AI

Knowledge-based AI aims to computationally model human knowledge by capturing concepts and knowledge used by individuals to solve problems or provide answers in specific domains. It relies on symbolic computing technologies to formalize and operationalize human knowledge into software.[11] A knowledge-based AI system works by utilizing AI techniques to store and organize knowledge in order to provide solutions, make decisions, or assist in problem-solving. The system typically uses a knowledge base, which is a repository of facts, rules, and information relevant to a specific domain. The knowledge is represented in the form of structured data, such as rules or facts, that can be used by the system to draw conclusions or make informed decisions.

Knowledge-based AI systems do have certain limitations that can affect their ability to leverage large volumes of data and automatically build knowledge models based on the data itself. Some of these limitations are:

- Reliance on existing knowledge: Knowledge-based AI systems rely heavily on pre-existing knowledge that is manually encoded into the system's knowledge base. This knowledge is typically created by human experts, and the process of authoring and maintaining this knowledge can be time-consuming and costly. This can limit the system's ability to adapt to new or evolving information, as it requires human intervention to update the knowledge base.

- Limited data-driven learning: Unlike data-driven AI systems such as machine learning, knowledge-based AI systems do not have the inherent ability to automatically learn from large volumes of data. They rely on explicitly defined rules and facts within the knowledge base to make decisions and draw conclusions. While knowledge-based systems can incorporate data, the process of integrating new data and updating the knowledge base often requires manual effort.

- Availability and accessibility of data: Knowledge-based AI systems may face challenges in accessing and utilizing large volumes of diverse data from various sources. The effectiveness of the system can be limited by the availability of relevant and reliable data that can be used to inform decision-making or enrich the knowledge base.

- High cost of knowledge authoring: The process of authoring and curating knowledge for knowledge-based AI systems can be resource-intensive and costly. It often requires domain experts to extract and encode their knowledge into the system's knowledge base. This can limit the scalability of knowledge-based systems and make it challenging to capture the breadth and depth of knowledge across multiple domains.

Data-driven AI

Data-driven AI, in the context of CDSS, involves using large amounts of human activity data stored in electronic patient records to extract patterns and insights for more effective outcomes in medical practice.[12] It employs statistical machine learning methods to analyze the data and make predictions, complete partial data, or emulate human behavior in similar conditions. This approach relies on big data and substantial computing power to achieve satisfactory performance levels.

For example, one application of data-driven AI in clinical practice is AI-enabled medical imaging analysis. Healthcare providers can utilize AI algorithms to analyze chest X-ray images and identify abnormalities or indicators of specific conditions like pneumonia or lung cancer. These algorithms use patterns and insights extracted from a large dataset of medical images to assist healthcare providers in making accurate diagnoses. By providing providers with AI-driven decision support, they can gain deeper insights into the analysis and improve their understanding of the AI-generated results.[13] Another relevant example is the use of AI algorithms in disease diagnosis. By making use of various medical data sources such as ultrasound, MRI, genomics, and computed tomography scans, AI techniques can assist healthcare providers in diagnosing diseases like Alzheimer's, cancer, diabetes, and heart disease more accurately.[14] These algorithms analyze patient data, identify patterns, and provide insights that aid in accurate and timely diagnosis.

To summarize, knowledge-based AI involves modeling human knowledge computationally and relies on top-down modeling from human self-reporting, while data-driven AI starts with large amounts of data and applies statistical machine learning methods to extract patterns for predictions and emulating human behavior. Data-driven AI requires access to big data and substantial computing power, while knowledge-based AI has limitations in leveraging large volumes of data and automatically building knowledge models based on the data itself, as well as potential constraints in evidence availability and high costs associated with human knowledge authoring processes. By combining the strengths of both knowledge-based and data-driven AI, researchers and practitioners can develop comprehensive CDSSs that leverage both human knowledge and large-scale clinical data, leading to more effective outcomes in practice.

Data acquisition and integration

CDSSs rely on the utilization of electronic medical records (EMRs) and other clinical data sources for data acquisition and integration.[2] These systems access and analyze data from various sources, including EMRs, laboratory results, imaging reports, and patient demographics, among others. The integration of these data sources enables CDSS to gather comprehensive patient information for decision-making purposes. Challenges and considerations in data acquisition for CDSS are also important to address. CDSS must ensure the availability, accuracy, and completeness of data from different sources.[15] Issues such as data interoperability, data quality, and data privacy need to be carefully managed to ensure the reliability and integrity of the information used by the system.

Knowledge representation and management

The creation of knowledge bases is a crucial component of clinical decision support.[16] In CDSS, knowledge bases refer to structured repositories of information that capture domain-specific knowledge and expertise. These knowledge bases are designed to support clinicians in their decision-making processes by providing relevant and evidence-based information at the point of care. The knowledge bases in CDSS systems contain various types of information, including clinical guidelines, medical literature, best practices, drug databases, patient data, and diagnostic criteria. They are organized and represented in a way that allows the CDSS to access and retrieve relevant information based on the specific context of a patient's condition.

The purpose of knowledge bases in CDSS systems is to enhance clinical decision-making by providing clinicians with timely and accurate information. When a clinician interacts with a CDSS, the system can query the knowledge base and retrieve relevant information to assist in diagnosing conditions, selecting appropriate treatments, identifying drug interactions, or providing recommendations for patient management. The knowledge bases in CDSS systems are continuously updated to incorporate the latest medical knowledge and research findings. They are often developed through a combination of manual knowledge authored by domain experts and automated methods for extracting and organizing information from medical literature and other sources.

By leveraging knowledge bases, CDSS systems can provide clinicians with evidence-based recommendations, reduce medical errors, improve adherence to guidelines, and enhance patient outcomes. However, it is important to ensure the quality and accuracy of the information stored in the knowledge bases to maintain the effectiveness and reliability of the CDSS. Machine learning and natural language processing techniques are also applied in CDSS for knowledge representation and management. Machine learning algorithms analyze patterns in patient data to identify associations, trends, and to make predictive models. Natural language processing techniques enable the system to extract meaningful information from unstructured medical text, such as clinical notes and research articles.

Decision support algorithms and models

CDSS utilizes various decision support algorithms and models to assist clinicians in their decision-making processes, including rule-based systems, Bayesian networks, neural networks, and clinical prediction models. Rule-based systems form a fundamental component of CDSS. These systems employ a set of predefined rules and logic to guide decision-making.[17] Rules are created based on medical guidelines, protocols, and expert knowledge. Rule-based systems provide clinicians with recommendations and alerts based on specific patient data and clinical conditions matched against the rule sets.

Bayesian networks play a significant role in decision support within CDSS.[18] These probabilistic models represent relationships between different medical variables and enable clinicians to assess the likelihood of certain outcomes. Bayesian networks use conditional probabilities to update probabilities based on new information, providing clinicians with insights into the probability of different diagnoses or treatment outcomes.

Neural networks and deep learning algorithms have gained prominence in CDSS.[19,20] These advanced models can analyze complex and high-dimensional patient data, such as medical images or genomic data, to support decision-making. Neural networks learn from these large datasets to recognize patterns and make predictions. Deep learning, a subset of neural networks, utilizes multiple layers of artificial neurons to extract intricate features from data, enabling more accurate predictions and risk assessments.

Clinical prediction models and risk stratification techniques are also employed in CDSS.[21,22] These models use patient data, such as demographics, medical history, and laboratory results, to estimate the probability of specific outcomes. Risk stratification models help identify patients at higher risk for certain conditions or adverse events, allowing clinicians to prioritize interventions and allocate resources effectively.

Advantages of AI in CDSS

Enhanced treatment recommendations and medication management

AI has a profound impact on treatment decision-making and medication optimization within CDSS. By leveraging large datasets and machine learning algorithms, CDSS can generate personalized treatment recommendations based on patient-specific factors such as medical history, genetics, and response to previous treatments. AI-powered CDSS can analyze enormous amounts of medical literature, clinical guidelines, and patient data to provide evidence-based treatment options tailored to individual patients. This capability ensures that clinicians have access to the most up-to-date information and can make informed decisions about appropriate treatment plans. Furthermore, AI in CDSS helps to optimize medication management by considering factors such as drug interactions, allergies, and patient characteristics, thereby reducing the risk of medication errors and adverse events. As an example, a systematic review, which analyzed 148 randomized controlled trials mainly involving adults, revealed that Clinical Decision Support (CDS) tools enhanced outcomes in several areas.[5] These improvements were noted in the delivery of preventive services (with an odds ratio [OR] of 1.42 and a 95% confidence interval [CI] of 1.27–1.58), in the ordering of clinical studies (OR of 1.72; 95% CI of 1.47–2.00), and in the prescribing of treatments (OR of 1.57; 95% CI of 1.35–1.82), compared to scenarios where CDS was not utilized.

Support for complex decision-making processes

AI plays a vital role in supporting healthcare providers in complex decision-making scenarios. CDSS equipped with AI algorithms can analyze and interpret complex datasets, integrating multiple variables and factors to provide comprehensive insights.[23,24] For example, in critical care settings, AI-powered CDSS can continuously monitor a patient's vital signs, laboratory results, and other clinical data to provide real-time decision support and predictive analytics.[25] This support aids clinicians in managing complex and dynamic patient conditions, identifying potential complications, and making timely interventions to optimize patient outcomes.

Timely alerts and reminders for critical situations

AI in CDSS contributes to the provision of timely alerts and reminders, especially in critical situations. CDSS can continuously monitor patient data, detect concerning trends or anomalies, and trigger alerts to notify healthcare providers of potential risks or urgent actions. AI-powered CDSS can alert healthcare providers about potential drug interactions, dosage errors, or critical changes in a patient's condition.[26] These timely alerts and reminders help to prevent medical errors, improve patient safety, and ensure that critical situations receive immediate attention. For example, researchers in Brigham and Women's Hospital showed that CDSS drug alerts reduced serious medication errors by 55%.[27]

Risks and challenges of AI in CDSS

Data-driven clinical support systems have several limitations that need to be considered.[15] These limitations can affect their effectiveness and impact on medical practice. Here are some key limitations of data-driven CSS:

- Quality and reliability of data: CDSS rely on large datasets, including electronic medical records, which can contain incomplete or inaccurate information. These data quality issues can lead to incorrect recommendations or decisions. The accuracy and reliability of data used in data-driven clinical support systems are crucial for generating meaningful insights. Issues such as missing data, data entry errors, and inconsistencies can affect the performance and reliability of these systems. Incomplete or erroneous data can lead to incorrect predictions or recommendations.
- Bias in data: Data-driven clinical support systems are susceptible to biases present in the data they rely on. If the data used to train these systems is biased, the resulting predictions or recommendations may also be biased, resulting in errors in treatment recommendations or diagnostic outcomes. Such biases can contribute to healthcare disparities and inequities if not properly addressed. Biases can arise from disparities in healthcare access, underrepresented patient populations, or variations in data collection practices. It is important to address and mitigate bias to ensure fair and equitable outcomes.
- Generalizability: Data-driven clinical support systems may struggle with generalizing findings to diverse patient populations. If the training data predominantly represents a specific demographic or

geographic region, the performance of the system may be limited when applied to different populations. Generalizability challenges can lead to suboptimal recommendations or predictions for underrepresented groups.

- Interpretability and explainability: Data-driven algorithms often operate as "black boxes," making it challenging to interpret and explain their decision-making processes. This lack of interpretability can undermine the trust and acceptance of these systems by clinicians and patients. There is a growing need for explainable AI techniques that provide transparent insights into how the system arrives at its predictions or recommendations.

- Ethical considerations: The integration of AI in CDSS raises ethical implications and privacy concerns. Ethical considerations arise when relying solely on AI algorithms for decision-making, as it may limit human autonomy and accountability. CDSS must strike a balance between providing support to healthcare professionals and allowing them to exercise their judgment based on ethical principles.

- Data privacy and security: Data-driven clinical support systems rely on sensitive patient information stored in EHRs. Ensuring the privacy and security of patient data is crucial to maintain trust and comply with privacy regulations. Any breaches or mishandling of patient data can have serious consequences for individuals and healthcare organizations. It is crucial to ensure robust data protection measures and adhere to relevant privacy regulations to safeguard patient confidentiality and prevent unauthorized access or misuse of data.

- Integration into clinical workflow: Integrating data-driven clinical support systems into existing clinical workflows can be challenging. These systems should seamlessly integrate with electronic medical records and other healthcare IT systems to provide real-time decision support without disrupting clinical operations. CDSS can disrupt a clinician's workflow, which can lead to increased cognitive effort, increased time to complete tasks, and less time spent with patients. Workflow integration requires careful planning, training, and change management to ensure successful adoption by healthcare professionals.

- Alert fatigue: Alert fatigue is a phenomenon that occurs when health-care professionals become desensitized after dealing with an overwhelming number of alerts.[28] Studies have shown that, in some systems, up to 95% of CDSS alerts are inconsequential.[29] As a result, health professionals may start to have slower response times to alert, and therefore may overlook or ignore them completely. For example, one study of drug alerts in the primary care setting demonstrated a decline in the utilization of an alert-based CDS with additional reminders for the same patient.[68]
- Interoperability issues in CDSS refer to challenges related to the seamless exchange and integration of information between different healthcare systems and components. Here is an overview of interoperability issues in CDSS:
  - Integration with EHR: CDSSs often rely on access to patient data stored in EHR systems. However, interoperability issues can arise when attempting to integrate CDSS with different EHR platforms that use different data formats, standards, or interfaces.[30] Incompatibilities between systems can hinder the smooth flow of information and limit the effectiveness of CDSS in utilizing comprehensive patient data.
  - Standardization of clinical data: CDSSs require access to standardized and structured clinical data for accurate decision support.[31] However, healthcare organizations may use different coding systems, terminologies, or data models, which can hinder interoperability. A lack of standardized clinical data across different systems can impede the integration of CDSS and limit their ability to provide consistent and meaningful decision support.
  - Data exchange between CDSS and other systems: CDSS may need to exchange data with various other healthcare systems, such as laboratory information systems, radiology systems, or pharmacy systems. Interoperability challenges can arise when there are discrepancies in data formats, protocols, or connectivity between these systems. Inconsistent data exchange mechanisms can hinder the timely and accurate delivery of information to support clinical decision-making.[32]
  - Semantic interoperability: Semantic interoperability refers to the ability of computer systems to exchange data with unambiguous,

shared meaning. In the context of CDSS, semantic interoperability enables seamless integration and processing of health data from diverse sources to provide accurate and timely decision recommendations.[33] As an example, suppose a patient moves from one healthcare provider to another. The patient's medical history, including diagnoses, treatments, and allergies, is stored in the EHR system of the first provider, which uses SNOMED CT for coding medical conditions. When the patient's records are transferred to the new provider's EHR system, semantic interoperability plays a crucial role. Even if the new provider uses a different EHR system, the use of SNOMED CT ensures that the diagnoses and treatments are interpreted accurately. Ensuring semantic interoperability is crucial for effective CDSS integration. This involves establishing a shared understanding and interpretation of clinical data across different systems. Semantic interoperability challenges can arise due to variations in terminology usage, differing interpretations of data elements, or inconsistent representation of clinical concepts.[34] Addressing these challenges is essential to enable accurate and meaningful decision support.

o   System compatibility and updates: CDSS must be compatible with the existing healthcare IT infrastructure, including hardware, operating systems, and network configurations. Interoperability issues can arise if CDSS software is not compatible with the technology stack used by healthcare organizations.[35] Additionally, as systems evolve and undergo updates or upgrades, compatibility issues can emerge, requiring careful coordination and testing to ensure smooth interoperability.

Addressing interoperability issues in CDSS requires collaborative efforts from healthcare organizations, standardization bodies, and technology providers. Developing and adopting interoperability standards, such as HL7 FHIR (Fast Healthcare Interoperability Resources), promoting data harmonization, and ensuring compatibility between different systems can help overcome these challenges and enable effective integration and utilization of CDSS in healthcare settings.

Usability issues

Usability refers to the ease of use and learnability of an interface design. A highly usable interface enables users to accomplish tasks, remember how to use the interface after periods of non-use, feel subjectively satisfied, and avoid or recover from errors quickly and efficiently.[36] Usability is therefore assessed by measuring factors such as the time required to learn the interface, speed of task completion, rate of errors made, user satisfaction ratings, and ease of re-establishing proficiency. The usability of AI-powered CDSS is a significant challenge, especially in terms of providing healthcare professionals with intuitive interfaces and user-friendly systems. When AI-powered CDSS lacks usability, it can result in resistance from healthcare professionals or suboptimal utilization of the technology, ultimately limiting the potential benefits that AI can provide in healthcare settings.[37] For example, if a CDSS interface is overly complex or difficult to navigate, healthcare providers may find it challenging to integrate the system into their workflow effectively. This could lead to frustration, resistance, or even abandonment of the CDSS, preventing them from fully leveraging its decision-support capabilities. Similarly, if the output or recommendations generated by an AI-powered CDSS are not presented in a clear and easily understandable manner, clinicians may struggle to interpret or trust the system's output. They might hesitate to rely on the CDSS for critical decision-making due to concerns about the accuracy, reliability, or relevance of the information provided. Furthermore, if the integration of AI-powered CDSS with existing healthcare systems is not seamless or requires excessive effort, healthcare providers may be deterred from adopting and utilizing the system. For example, if the CDSS requires extensive data entry or manual input of patient information, clinicians may find it time-consuming or burdensome, leading to reduced usage or limited integration of the system into their practice. Addressing the usability challenges of AI-powered CDSS requires careful consideration of the user experience, user interface design, and workflow integration. By involving physicians and other end-users in the design and development process, CDSS can be tailored to meet their needs and preferences, making it more intuitive and user-friendly. Additionally, providing comprehensive training, ongoing support, and feedback mechanisms can help healthcare professionals better understand and embrace the capabilities of AI-powered CDSS, leading to improved utilization and ultimately enhancing patient care outcomes. The usability of AI-powered CDSS is another challenge, as healthcare professionals need intuitive interfaces and user-friendly systems to efficiently utilize the technology. Poor system usability can lead to resistance or suboptimal utilization, limiting the benefits AI can provide.

Impact on provider workflow and decision-making

The introduction of AI in CDSS can have significant implications for healthcare professionals' workflow and decision-making processes. The reliance on AI algorithms for decision support may disrupt established workflows, requiring healthcare professionals to adapt to new processes and incorporate AI-generated recommendations into their practice.[38,39] This adjustment period can result in resistance, skepticism, or even mistrust toward AI systems. Additionally, healthcare professionals need to understand the underlying logic and reasoning of AI algorithms to confidently trust and interpret their outputs. Transparent and explainable AI models are necessary for building trust and facilitating effective collaboration between AI and healthcare professionals.

The impact of professional deskilling as AI Systems are introduced into the healthcare system

Since the early twentieth century, job design within enterprises has followed a trend toward decreased worker skill requirements, known as "deskilling." This historical pattern emerged as production shifted from small craft-based shops to large factories. Influential thinkers like Adam Smith (1776) and Charles Babbage (1835) promoted the idea of dividing labor into specialized tasks and roles to increase efficiency. Frederick Winslow Taylor (1911) built on this notion through his principles of scientific management, which prescribed standardized processes with narrow, simplified job duties. The widespread adoption of assembly lines enabled mass production, with each worker focusing on a single, repetitive task. Between the rise of industrial factories, influential philosophical ideas, and engineered management practices, jobs transformed from skilled artisans producing whole products to low-skilled workers carrying out limited, predefined tasks in a segmented production sequence. In many modern industries, this early twentieth century trend toward simplification and deskilling of jobs remains influential in how roles are designed today. By breaking down jobs into minimal skill sets and narrow duties, enterprises have been able to maximize efficiency and output, while minimizing required training. However, some experts argue this has reduced opportunities for skill development and creativity among individual workers. Professional deskilling in the context of AI implementation in healthcare refers to the loss or reduction in the skill set and expertise of healthcare professionals as certain tasks or responsibilities are automated or delegated to AI systems. As AI technology advances, there is a possibility that routine or standardized healthcare tasks, such as diagnosis, treatment planning, and data analysis, can be performed more efficiently and accurately by AI algorithms. This can lead to a shift in the division of labor, with AI taking over certain aspects of healthcare decision-making traditionally performed by professionals.

AI systems have the potential to augment healthcare professionals by assisting in diagnosis, treatment planning, and decision-making. However, concerns arise when AI is perceived as a replacement for healthcare professionals, leading to the potential erosion of their expertise and clinical judgment. Striking the right balance between human expertise and AI assistance is crucial. Overreliance on AI-generated outputs without critical assessment and validation by healthcare professionals can lead to the erosion of their clinical skills.[40] If healthcare professionals rely heavily on AI interpretations without independently verifying them, there is a risk of diminished proficiency in their own diagnostic and decision-making abilities. As AI algorithms become more proficient in interpreting medical data, healthcare professionals may gradually lose their interpretive skills in specific areas. For example, in specialties like radiology or pathology, where AI has shown significant advancements, there is a potential risk of diminished expertise if professionals rely solely on AI interpretations. The concept of professional de-skilling raises concerns about the impact on healthcare professionals, particularly their job roles, job satisfaction, and the overall quality of care provided. It is essential to carefully navigate the implementation of AI in healthcare to ensure that professionals are not marginalized or replaced by AI systems but rather empowered to collaborate effectively with these technologies.

Impact of alert fatigue

Alert fatigue in medicine refers to the phenomenon where healthcare professionals become desensitized or overwhelmed by the high volume of clinical alerts and notifications generated by EHR systems, medical devices, and other healthcare technologies.[41] These alerts are designed to provide timely information about patient conditions, test results, medication orders, and potential safety issues.[42] However, with the increasing adoption of health information technology, healthcare providers are faced with an abundance of alerts, many of which may be non-critical or irrelevant.[43] As a result, they may start to ignore or dismiss alerts, even those that are clinically significant, leading to a potential increase in medical errors and patient safety risks.[44] Alert fatigue can have serious implications for patient care and safety. When healthcare professionals are inundated with numerous low-value or non-actionable alerts, they may miss important alerts or fail to respond promptly to critical situations. Indeed, some studies report overriding rates ranging between 77% and 90%.[45-47] This can result in delayed diagnosis, medication errors, or overlooking vital patient information, potentially compromising patient outcomes.

Future trends in CDSS

The future of CDSS is bright and filled with exciting possibilities. Advancements in natural language processing, integration of genomics and personalized medicine, and clinical decision support in remote settings are shaping the landscape of CDSS. As we navigate these emerging trends, it is crucial to strike a balance between technological advancements and ethical responsibility to harness the full potential of CDSS for improving patient outcomes and healthcare delivery.

Advancements in natural language processing and clinical language understanding

Natural language processing (NLP) is a field of AI that enables computers to understand, interpret, and generate human language. NLP focuses on developing algorithms and models that can automatically analyze text and speech to extract key information. This includes tasks like translation, sentiment analysis, speech recognition, and text summarization. The overarching goal of NLP is to teach machines to comprehend and respond to natural human communication and language, not just structured data. An NLP system takes in unstructured human language as input, applies analytical algorithms to it, and produces structured data or natural language output that responds appropriately to the input. By enabling computers to synthesize and extract meaning from human language, NLP aims to support seamless human-computer interaction through natural communication. NLP can also allow CDSS to extract and analyze meaningful information from unstructured clinical text, including medical notes and research articles.[48] By unlocking insights from this enormous amount of data, NLP enhances the capabilities of CDSS and enables more informed decision-making.

- Improved information extraction: NLP techniques facilitate the extraction of relevant information from unstructured clinical text.[49] For example, NLP algorithms can identify patient demographics, medical conditions, procedures, medications, and laboratory results from EHRs.[50] This information extraction allows CDSS to access critical data for generating tailored recommendations and alerts.
- Clinical concept recognition: NLP algorithms enable the recognition and understanding of clinical concepts within the text. This involves identifying medical terms, anatomical entities, symptoms, and other relevant information. By accurately recognizing these concepts, CDSS can interpret and process the text effectively. For instance, NLP can recognize that "chest pain" and "angina" refer to the same clinical concept, enabling more accurate analysis and decision support.

- Semantic understanding: NLP goes beyond simple keyword matching by understanding the meaning and context of the text. Through semantic understanding, NLP algorithms can grasp the relationships between words and phrases. This capability allows CDSS to capture the nuances of clinical information and generate more contextually relevant recommendations. For example, NLP can interpret "patient has a history of heart attack," which implies a higher risk for cardio-vascular events and hence, provide appropriate decision support.

NLP is applied in various ways to enhance CDSS. One example is extracting pertinent patient information from EHRs. NLP algorithms can automatically identify relevant clinical data, such as diagnoses, treat-ments, and medications, thereby saving time for healthcare providers and ensuring accurate and up-to-date information for decision support. Additionally, NLP improves clinical documentation accuracy by auto-matically suggesting standardized terminology and identifying inconsist-encies or missing information in clinical notes. Another application is clinical research, where NLP enables the extraction of valuable insights from medical literature. NLP algorithms can analyze research articles to identify relevant evidence, treatment guidelines, and clinical trials. This helps CDSS stay updated with the latest medical knowledge and provide evidence-based recommendations.

Integration of genomics and personalized medicine in CDSS

The integration of genomics and personalized medicine presents a promis-ing future for CDSS.[51] By leveraging genetic information, CDSS can predict disease risk, guide treatment selection, and optimize medication dosages for individual patients, ultimately enhancing patient care outcomes.

- Predicting disease risk: Genomic data provides valuable insights into an individual's predisposition to certain diseases. CDSS can utilize genetic markers and variations to assess a patient's genetic risk profile and identify their susceptibility to specific conditions.[52] For example, by analyzing genetic information, CDSS can predict the likelihood of developing diseases such as cardiovascular disorders, and certain cancers, and hereditary conditions like familial hypercholesterolemia. Armed with this knowledge, healthcare providers can implement preventive measures and tailor screening strategies for high-risk patients, leading to early detection and improved outcomes.

- Guiding treatment selection: An individual's genetic makeup can affect how their body processes and responds to certain medications. Variations in a person's genes influence the activity of proteins involved in drug metabolism, transportation, and receptor binding. This means some genetic variants may cause a drug to be broken down faster or slower, impact how it is absorbed and circulated, or alter its ability to bind to targets. As a result, the drug may exhibit reduced efficacy or increased toxicity in people with certain genotypes. Pharmacogenetic testing helps to identify genetic factors that contribute to changes in drug effects between individuals, enabling more personalized medication selection and dosing.[53] Genomic data can guide treatment decisions by offering personalized recommendations based on an individual's genetic profile. CDSS can analyze genetic variations that influence drug response and metabolism to identify the most effective treatment options.[54] For instance, certain genetic markers can indicate a patient's likelihood of responding to specific medications or experiencing adverse drug reactions.[69] CDSS can provide recommendations tailored to the patient's genetic makeup, helping clinicians choose the most suitable therapies and avoid potentially harmful interventions.

- Optimizing medication dosages: Personalized medicine considers an individual's genetic factors when determining optimal medication dosages. CDSS can incorporate genomic data to calculate the precise dosage requirements based on genetic variations that affect drug metabolism and response.[55] By considering a patient's genetic profile, CDSS can minimize the risk of under or overmedication, improving treatment efficacy and reducing adverse effects. For example, in the field of oncology, CDSS can leverage genomic data to determine the ideal dosage of chemotherapy drugs based on a patient's genetic markers, ensuring tailored treatment plans and better therapeutic outcomes.[70]

Genomics and personalized medicine have already showcased their potential in CDSS. For instance, pharmacogenomics, which examines the relationship between an individual's genetic makeup and drug response, has been integrated into CDSS. By analyzing genetic variations in drug-metabolizing enzymes, CDSS can identify patients who are at higher risk for adverse drug reactions or those who may require dosage adjustments for certain medications. This empowers clinicians to make informed decisions regarding medication selection and dosing, enhancing patient safety and treatment outcomes. Another example is the development of targeted therapies based on an individual's genomic profile. CDSS can analyze genetic alterations or mutations in tumor cells to identify specific molecular targets for therapy.[56] This enables the selection of precise treatment options, such as targeted therapies or immunotherapies, tailored to the patient's unique genetic characteristics. By integrating genomics into CDSS, healthcare providers can offer personalized treatment strategies, leading to more effective interventions and improved patient outcomes.

Clinical decision support for remote and telemedicine settings

The rapid expansion of remote healthcare and telemedicine has created new avenues for the application of CDSS, including enabling virtual consultations, remote monitoring, and point-of-care decision support.[57]

- Enabling virtual consultations: CDSS plays a vital role in facilitating virtual consultations between healthcare providers and patients.[58] Through video conferencing or teleconferencing platforms, CDSS provides decision support by analyzing patient data in real-time. For example, during a virtual consultation, CDSS can integrate patient information from EHRs, remote monitoring devices, and patient-reported data to provide clinicians with immediate insights, assist in diagnosis, and offer treatment recommendations.[71] This enhances the quality of remote healthcare delivery and ensures that patients receive timely and accurate care.

- Remote monitoring: CDSS enables remote monitoring of patients' health conditions and can alert healthcare providers to potential issues.[59] By integrating data from wearable devices, sensors, and remote monitoring technologies, CDSS can continuously analyze patient data and provide alerts or notifications for critical events. For instance, in cases of chronic diseases like diabetes or hypertension, CDSS can track vital signs, blood glucose levels, or medication adherence. If any anomalies or deviations from the expected range occur, CDSS can promptly alert healthcare providers, allowing for timely intervention and improved patient outcomes.

- Decision support at the point of care: CDSS brings decision support capabilities directly to the point of care in remote settings.[60-62] Through AI algorithms, CDSS can analyze patient data in real-time and provide evidence-based recommendations to healthcare providers. For instance, during a remote consultation, CDSS can assist with medication selection, dosage calculations, or treatment guidelines based on the patient's condition, medical history, and real-time data.[72] This ensures that healthcare providers have the necessary support and guidance to make informed decisions, even in remote settings.

Challenges and opportunities

Implementing CDSS in telemedicine presents both challenges and opportunities. One challenge is ensuring reliable data transmission and connectivity, especially in areas with limited internet access or unstable networks.[63] Additionally, remote access to patient records and integration of diverse data sources can pose technical hurdles that need to be addressed. Furthermore, maintaining patient privacy and data security is of utmost importance.[64] CDSS must comply with privacy regulations and adopt robust security measures to protect sensitive patient information during remote consultations.

CDSS in telemedicine has already demonstrated its effectiveness in various scenarios. For example, AI-powered virtual assistants, such as chatbots or voice assistants, can be utilized to provide real-time guidance to healthcare providers during remote consultations. These virtual assistants can analyze patient data, offer treatment suggestions, and answer questions based on clinical guidelines and best practices.[65] They serve as valuable tools that enhance the efficiency and effectiveness of remote healthcare delivery, particularly in resource-constrained settings. Furthermore, remote monitoring solutions that leverage CDSS have been successfully implemented. For instance, in the management of chronic conditions like heart failure, CDSS can analyze data from implantable devices, such as pacemakers or defibrillators, and alert healthcare providers to changes in a patient's condition.[66] This allows for early intervention and reduces the risk of complications.

Conclusion

The integration of Clinical Decision Support Systems (CDSS) with the power of AI has proven to be a game-changer in healthcare. This chapter has explored the various aspects of CDSS and highlighted the transformative role that AI plays in improving clinical decision-making and patient outcomes. By harnessing the vast amounts of data available in EHRs, medical literature, and patient-generated information, AI-driven CDSS has the potential to revolutionize healthcare delivery.

The use of AI in CDSS brings a multitude of benefits to clinical decision-making. AI algorithms can quickly analyze and interpret complex data, identifying patterns and generating insights that may elude human practitioners. Through machine learning, AI models continuously learn and adapt to new data, improving their accuracy and effectiveness over time. This dynamic and evolving nature of AI ensures that CDSS remains up-to-date with the latest medical knowledge and evidence-based practices. The impact of AI-driven CDSS on patient outcomes cannot be overstated. By providing clinicians with timely, evidence-based recommendations and alerts, CDSS helps reduce diagnostic errors, improve treatment selection, and optimize medication management. Real-time access to relevant patient data, integrated seamlessly into the clinical workflow, enables healthcare providers to make informed decisions at the point of care. This leads to more personalized and precise interventions, ultimately resulting in enhanced patient safety, improved health outcomes, and increased patient satisfaction.

Moreover, AI-driven CDSS has the potential to address healthcare disparities by reducing variability in clinical practice. By integrating standardized guidelines and best practices, CDSS ensures that patients receive consistent, high-quality care regardless of the individual clinician's experience or expertise. This promotes healthcare equity and contributes to a more efficient and effective healthcare system.

However, the successful implementation of AI-driven CDSS requires careful consideration of ethical and regulatory considerations. Safeguarding patient privacy, ensuring data security, and maintaining transparency and accountability in algorithmic decision-making are critical aspects that must be addressed. Collaboration between clinicians, data scientists, and policymakers is essential to establish guidelines and frameworks that uphold ethical standards and maximize the potential benefits of AI in CDSS.

References

1. Osheroff JA, Teich JM, Middleton B, Steen EB, Wright A, Detmer DE. (2007) A roadmap for national action on clinical decision support. *Journal of the American Medical Informatics Association*, **14**(2), 141–145. Erratum in: *Journal of the American Medical Informatics Association*, **14**(3), 389.
2. Berner ES, La Lande TJ. (2016) Overview of clinical decision support systems. In *Clinical Decision Support Systems: Theory and Practice, 3rd edition*, Berner ES (ed.), New York, Springer, 3–22.
3. Adams R, Henry KE, Sridharan A, *et al.* (2022) Prospective, multi-site study of patient outcomes after implementation of the TREWS machine learning-based early warning system for sepsis. *Nature Medicine*, **28**, 1455–1460.
4. Garg AX, Adhikari NK, McDonald H, Rosas-Arellano MP, Devereaux PJ, Beyene J, Sam J, Haynes RB. (2005) Effects of computerized clinical decision support systems on practitioner performance and patient outcomes: a systematic review. *JAMA Network*, **293**(10), 1223–1238.
5. Bright TJ, Wong A, Dhurjati R, Bristow E, Bastian L, Coeytaux RR, Samsa G, Hasselblad V, Williams JW, Musty MD, Wing L, Kendrick AS, Sanders

GD, Lobach D. (2012) Effect of clinical decision-support systems: a systematic review. *Annals of Internal Medicine*, **157**(1), 29–43.

6. Kawamoto K, Houlihan CA, Balas EA, Lobach DF. (2005) Improving clinical practice using clinical decision support systems: a systematic review of trials to identify features critical to success. *BMJ*, **330**(7494), 765.

7. McGinn TG, McCullagh L, Kannry J, Knaus M, Sofianou A, Wisnivesky JP, Mann DM. (2013) Efficacy of an evidence-based clinical decision support in primary care practices: a randomized clinical trial. *JAMA Internal Medicine*, **173**(17), 1584–1591.

8. Shortliffe EH. (1987) Computer programs to support clinical decision making. *JAMA Network*, **258**(1), 61–66.

9. Goodman KE, Morgan DJ, Hoffmann DE. (2023) Clinical algorithms, antidiscrimination laws, and medical device regulation. *JAMA Network*, **329**, 285–286.

10. Blumenthal D, Tavenner M. (2010) The "meaningful use" regulation for electronic health records. *The New England Journal of Medicine*, **363**(6), 501–504.

11. Patel VL, Shortliffe EH, Stefanelli M, Szolovits P, Berthold MR, Bellazzi R, Abu-Hanna A. (2009) The coming of age of artificial intelligence in medicine. *Artificial Intelligence in Medicine*, **46**(1), 5–17.

12. Chen JH, Asch SM. Machine learning and prediction in medicine — beyond the peak of inflated expectations. *The New England Journal of Medicine*, **376**(26), 2507–2509.

13. Cai CJ, Winter S, Steiner D, Wilcox L, Terry M. (2019) "Hello AI": uncovering the onboarding needs of medical practitioners for human-AI collaborative decision-making. *Proceedings of the ACM on Human-Computer Interaction*, **3**(CSCW), 1–24.

14. Jiang F, Jiang Y, Zhi H, Dong Y, Li H, Ma S, Wang Y, Dong Q, Shen H, Wang Y. (2017) Artificial intelligence in healthcare: past, present and future. *Stroke and Vascular Neurology*, **2**(4), 230–243.

15. Kuperman GJ, Bobb A, Payne TH, Avery AJ, Gandhi TK, Burns G, Classen DC, Bates DW. (2007) Medication-related clinical decision support in computerized provider order entry systems: a review. *Journal of the American Medical Informatics Association*, **14**(1), 29–40.

16. Müller L, Gangadharaiah R, Klein SC, *et al.* (2019) An open access medical knowledge base for community driven diagnostic decision support system development. *BMC Medical Informatics and Decision Making*, **19**, 93.

17. Sutton RT, Pincock D, Baumgart DC, Sadowski DC, Fedorak RN, Kroeker KI. (2020) An overview of clinical decision support systems: benefits, risks, and strategies for success. *npj Digital Medicine*, **3**, 17.
18. Sesen MB, Nicholson AE, Banares-Alcantara R, Kadir T, Brady M. (2013) Bayesian networks for clinical decision support in lung cancer care. *PLoS One*, **8**(12), e82349.
19. McCullum N. (2020) Deep learning neural networks explained in plain English. https://www.freecodecamp.org/news/deep-learning-neural-networks-explained-in-plain-english/
20. Ahsan MM, Luna SA, Siddique Z. (2022) Machine-learning-based disease diagnosis: a comprehensive review. *Healthcare (Basel)*, **10**(3), 541.
21. Stagg BC, Stein JD, Medeiros FA, Wirostko B, Crandall A, Hartnett ME, Cummins M, Morris A, Hess R, Kawamoto K. (2021) Special commentary: using clinical decision support systems to bring predictive models to the glaucoma clinic. *Ophthalmology Glaucoma*, **4**(1), 5–9.
22. Choi GH, Yun J, Choi J, *et al.* (2020) Development of machine learning-based clinical decision support system for hepatocellular carcinoma. *Scientific Reports*, **10**, 14855.
23. Komorowski M, Celi LA, Badawi O, Gordon AC, Faisal AA. (2018) The artificial intelligence clinician learns optimal treatment strategies for sepsis in intensive care. *Nature Medicine*, **24**(11), 1716–1720.
24. Jalalian A, Mashohor SB, Mahmud HR, Saripan MI, Ramli AR, Karasfi B. (20130 Computer-aided detection/diagnosis of breast cancer in mammography and ultrasound: a review. Clinical Imaging, **37**(3), 420–426.
25. Johnson A, Ghassemi M, *et al.* (2016) Machine learning and decision support in critical care. *Proceedings of the IEEE*, **104**(2), 444–466.
26. Cho KJ, Kwon O, Kwon JM, Lee Y, Park H, Jeon KH, Kim KH, Park J, Oh BH. (2020) Detecting patient deterioration using artificial intelligence in a rapid response system. *Critical Care Medicine*, **48**(4), e285–e289.
27. Kaushal R, Shojania KG, Bates DW. (2003) Effects of computerized physician order entry and clinical decision support systems on medication safety: a systematic review. *Arch Intern Med*, **163**(12), 1409–1416.
28. Khalifa M, Zabani I. (2016) Improving utilization of clinical decision support systems by reducing alert fatigue: strategies and recommendations. *Studies in Health Technology and Informatics*, **226**, 51–54.
29. Ash JS, Sittig DF, Campbell EM, Guappone KP, Dykstra RH. (2007) Some unintended consequences of clinical decision support systems. *AMIA Annual Symposium Proceedings, AMIA Symposium*, **2007**, 26–30.

30. Edwards A, Hollin I, Barry J, Kachnowski S. (2010) Barriers to cross--institutional health information exchange: a literature review. *Health Information Management Journal*, **24**(3), 22–34.

31. Jia P, Zhao P, Chen J, Zhang M. (2019) Evaluation of clinical decision support systems for diabetes care: An overview of current evidence. *Journal of Evaluation in Clinical Practice*, **25**(1), 66–77.

32. Stone EG. (2018) Unintended adverse consequences of a clinical decision support system: two cases. *Journal of the American Medical Informatics Association*, **25**(5), 564–567.

33. de Mello BH, Rigo SJ, da Costa CA, da Rosa Righi R, Donida B, Bez MR, Schunke LC. (2022) Semantic interoperability in health records standards: a systematic literature review. Health Technology (Berl), **12**(2), 255–272.

34. Kim D-Y, Joshi KP. (2021) A semantically rich knowledge graph to automate HIPAA regulations for Cloud Health IT services. https://ebiquity.umbc.edu/paper/html/id/976/A-Semantically-Rich-Knowledge-Graph-to-Automate-HIPAA-Regulations-for-Cloud-Health-IT-Services

35. Marcos M, Maldonado JA, Martínez-Salvador B, Boscá D, Robles M. (2013) Interoperability of clinical decision-support systems and electronic health records using archetypes: a case study in clinical trial eligibility. *Journal of Biomedical Informatics*, **46**(4), 676–689.

36. Nielsen J. Usability 101: introduction to usability. (2012) https://www.nngroup.com/articles/usability-101-introduction-to-usability/

37. Genes N, Kim MS, Thum FL, Rivera L, Beato R, Song C, Soriano J, Kannry J, Baumlin K, Hwang U. (2016) Usability evaluation of a clinical decision support system for geriatric ED pain treatment. *Applied Clinical Informatics*, **7**(1), 128–142.

38. Olakotan OO, Mohd Yusof M. (2021) The appropriateness of clinical decision support systems alerts in supporting clinical workflows: a systematic review. *Health Informatics Journal*, **27**(2), 14604582211007536.

39. Sittig DF, Wright A, Osheroff JA, *et al.* (2008) Grand challenges in clinical decision support. *Journal of Biomedical Informatics*, **41**(2), 387–392.

40. Alami H, Gagnon MP, Fortin JP. (2019) Some multidimensional unintended consequences of telehealth utilization: a multi-project evaluation synthesis. *International Journal of Health Policy and Management*, **8**(6), 337–352.

41. Van DSH. (2016) Errors related to alert fatigue. In *Safety of Health IT*, Agrawal A (ed.), Springer, Cham, 41–54.

42. Kamel Boulos MN, Wilson JT, Clauson KA. (2018) Geospatial blockchain: promises, challenges, and scenarios in health and healthcare. *International Journal of Health Geographics*, **17**(1), 25.

43. Chien S-C, Chin Y-P, Yoon CH, Islam MM, Jian W-S, Hsu C-K, Chen C-Y, Chien P-H, Li Y-C. (2021) A novel method to retrieve alerts from a home-grown Computerized Physician Order Entry (CPOE) system of an academic medical center: comprehensive alert characteristic analysis. *PLoS ONE*, **16**, e0246597.

44. Rayo MF, Kowalczyk N, Liston BW, Sanders EB, White S, Patterson ES. (2015) Comparing the effectiveness of alerts and Dynamically Annotated Visualizations (DAVs) in improving clinical decision making. *Human Factors*, **57**(6), 1002–1014.

45. McGreevey JD, Mallozzi CP, Perkins RM, Shelov E, Schreiber R. (2020) Reducing alert burden in electronic health records: state of the art recommendations from four health systems. *Applied Clinical Informatics*, **11**(1), 1–12.

46. Isaac T, Weissman JS, Davis RB, Massagli M, Cyrulik A, Sands DZ, *et al.* (2009) Overrides of medication alerts in ambulatory care. *Arch Intern Med*, **169**(3), 305–311.

47. van DSH, Aarts J, Vulto A, Berg M. (2006) Overriding of drug safety alerts in computerized physician order entry. *Journal of the American Medical Informatics Association*, **13**(2), 138–147.

48. (2018) The use of NLP to extract unstructured medical data from text. https://insidebigdata.com/2018/09/03/use-nlp-extract-unstructured-medical-data-text/

49. BuHamra SS, Almutairi AN, Buhamrah AK, Almadani SH, Alibrahim YA. (2022) An NLP tool for data extraction from electronic health records: COVID-19 mortalities and comorbidities. *Frontiers in Public Health*, **10**, 1070870.

50. Spasić I, Uzuner O, Zhou L. (2020) Emerging clinical applications of text analytics. *International Journal of Medical Informatics*, **134**, 103974.

51. Overby CL, Kohane I, Kannry JL, Williams MS, Starren J, Bottinger E, Gottesman O, Denny JC, Weng C, Tarczy-Hornoch P, Hripcsak G. (2013) Opportunities for genomic clinical decision support interventions. *Genetics in Medicine*, **15**(10), 817–823.

52. Welch BM, Kawamoto K. (2013) Clinical decision support for genetically guided personalized medicine: a systematic review. *Journal of the American Medical Informatics Association*, **20**(2), 388–400.

53. Stanek EJ, Sanders CL, Taber KA, *et al.* (2012) Adoption of pharmacogenomic testing by US physicians: results of a nationwide survey. *Clinical Pharmacology & Therapeutics*, **91**(3), 450–458.

54. Hinderer M, Boeker M, Wagner SA, Lablans M, Newe S, Hülsemann JL, Neumaier M, Binder H, Renz H, Acker T, Prokosch HU, Sedlmayr M. (2017) Integrating clinical decision support systems for pharmacogenomic testing into clinical routine — a scoping review of designs of user-system interactions in recent system development. *BMC Medical Informatics and Decision Making*, **17**(1), 81.

55. Pavani A, Naushad SM, Kumar RM , Srinath M, Malempati AR, Kutala VK. (2016) Artificial neural network-based pharmacogenomic algorithm for warfarin dose optimization. *Pharmacogenomics*, **17**, 121–131.

56. Tamborero D, Dienstmann R, Rachid MH, Boekel J, Lopez-Fernandez A, Jonsson M, Razzak A, Braña I, De Petris L, Yachnin J, Baird RD, Loriot Y, Massard C, Martin-Romano P, Opdam F, Schlenk RF, Vernieri C, Masucci M, Villalobos X, Chavarria E; Cancer Core Europe consortium; Balmaña J, Apolone G, Caldas C, Bergh J, Ernberg I, Fröhling S, Garralda E, Karlsson C, Tabernero J, Voest E, Rodon J, Lehtiö J. (2022) The Molecular Tumor Board Portal supports clinical decisions and automated reporting for precision oncology. *Nature Cancer*, **3**(2), 251–261. Erratum in: *Nature Cancer*, **3**(5), 649.

57. Wiwatkunupakarn N, Aramrat C, Pliannuom S, Buawangpong N, Pinyopornpanish K, Nantsupawat N, Mallinson PAC, Kinra S, Angkurawaranon C. (2023) The integration of clinical decision support systems into telemedicine for patients with multimorbidity in primary care settings: scoping review. *Journal of Medical Internet Research*, **25**, e45944.

58. Atta-ur-Rahman, Ahmed MIB. (2019) Chapter 15 — Virtual Clinic: A CDSS Assisted Telemedicine Framework. In *Telemedicine Technologies*, Jude HD, Balas VE (eds.), Academic Press, 227–238.

59. Shanmathi N, Jagannath M. (2018) Computerized decision support system for remote health monitoring: a systematic review. *IRBM*, **39**(5), 359–367.

60. Agarwal S, Glenton C, Tamrat T, Henschke N, Maayan N, Fønhus MS, Mehl GL, Lewin S. (2021) Decision-support tools via mobile devices to improve quality of care in primary healthcare settings. *Cochrane Database of Systematic Reviews*, **7**(7), CD012944.

61. DSS Inc. Radiology Decision Support (RadWise®). https://www.dssinc.com/products/integrated-clinical-products/radwise-radiology-decision-support/

62. Embi PJ, Jain A, Clark J, Harris CM. (2005) Development of an electronic health record-based Clinical Trial Alert system to enhance recruitment at the point of care. *AMIA Annual Symposium Proceedings*, **2005**, 231–235.

63. Jefee-Bahloul H, Barkil-Oteo A, Augusterfer EF. (2017) *Telemental Health in Resource-Limited Global Setting*, Oxford, UK, Oxford University Press.

64. Ali N, Khalifa O, Abd Manaf A. (2013) ICT in telemedicine: conquering privacy and security issues in health care services. *Electronic Journal of Computer Science and Information Technology*, **4**(1).

65. Koulaouzidis G, Charisopoulou D, Wojakowski W, Koulaouzidis A, Marlicz W, Jadczyk T. (2020) Telemedicine in cardiology in the time of coronavirus disease 2019: a friend that everybody needs. *Polish Archives of Internal Medicine*, **130**(6), 559–561.

66. Guidi GP. (2015) A multi-layer monitoring system for clinical management of Congestive Heart Failure. *BMC Medical Informatics and Decision Making*, **15**, S5.

67. Ledley RS, Lusted LB. (1959) Reasoning foundations of medical diagnosis; symbolic logic, probability, and value theory aid our understanding of how physicians reason. *Science*, **130**, 9–21.

68. Ancker JS, *et al.* (2017) Effects of workload, work complexity, and repeated alerts on alert fatigue in a clinical decision support system. *BMC Medical Informatics and Decision Making*, **17**, 36.

69. Ventola CL. (2011) Pharmacogenomics in clinical practice: reality and expectations. *P & T: A Peer-reviewed Journal for Formulary Management*, **36**(7), 412–450.

70. Innocenti F, Cox NJ, Dolan ME. (2011) The use of genomic information to optimize cancer chemotherapy. *Seminars in Oncology*, **38**(2), 186–195.

71. Kristoffersson A, Coradeschi S, Loutfi A. (2013) A review of Mobile Robotic Telepresence. *Advances in Human-Computer Interaction*, **2013**, 902316, 17.

72. Surgical telepresence technology connects remote areas to world-class healthcare. https://medjournal360.com/internal-medicine/surgical-telepresence-technology-connects-remote-areas-to-world-class-healthcare/

Chapter 17

Collaborative Learning and Knowledge Sharing in AI-Driven Healthcare

Introduction

In the rapidly evolving landscape of AI-driven healthcare, the collaboration between healthcare professionals and artificial intelligence (AI) experts has become paramount.[1] The integration of AI and medicine holds immense potential for advancing patient care, improving decision-making processes, and accelerating innovation.[2,3] To harness the full power of this collaboration, fostering collaborative learning and knowledge sharing among healthcare professionals and AI experts is essential. This chapter explores the critical role of collaboration in AI-driven healthcare and examines the strategies for facilitating interdisciplinary research, training initiatives, and sharing best practices in the field. By promoting collaboration and knowledge exchange, healthcare professionals and AI experts can collectively shape the future of healthcare. Through this chapter, we aim to provide valuable insights into the importance of collaborative learning and knowledge sharing in the context of AI-driven healthcare.

Facilitating collaboration and knowledge exchange among healthcare professionals and AI experts

Facilitating collaboration and knowledge exchange among healthcare professionals and AI experts is vital for unlocking the full potential of AI-driven healthcare. This section will discuss the importance of collaboration between healthcare professionals and AI experts, highlighting both the benefits and challenges associated with this collaborative approach. Collaboration between healthcare professionals and AI experts offers numerous benefits that positively impact patient care and outcomes. Firstly, by working together, healthcare professionals can make more informed decisions by leveraging the analytical capabilities of AI systems. The integration of AI technologies can enhance diagnostic accuracy, treatment planning, and predictive modeling, ultimately leading to improved patient outcomes.[4] Moreover, collaboration enables the identification of novel solutions and approaches to complex healthcare problems, fostering accelerated innovation in the field. For example, collaboration between healthcare professionals and AI experts was instrumental in the field of cardiology. Awni Hannun, a computer scientist, and Geoffrey Tison, a cardiologist, and colleagues at Stanford University developed a deep neural network capable of detecting and classifying arrhythmias in ambulatory electrocardiograms.[5] The algorithm achieved performance comparable to cardiologists, highlighting the potential of AI in assisting in the diagnosis of cardiac conditions and the advantages of cross-collaboration.

However, collaboration between healthcare professionals and AI experts presents certain challenges that need to be addressed. Effective communication and understanding between the two groups are paramount to successful collaboration. Communication barriers arising from differences in professional language, perspectives, and knowledge domains must be overcome to ensure effective knowledge exchange. Additionally, the divergent perspectives between healthcare professionals and AI experts require mutual understanding and a shared vision for collaborative efforts to yield optimal results.[6]

As Schot and colleagues stated in their 2018 article in the Journal of Interprofessional Care,[7] professionals from different fields contribute to interprofessional collaboration by bridging professional, social, physical, and task-related gaps, negotiating overlaps in roles and tasks, and creating spaces to facilitate such collaboration. Each profession brings unique contributions to the collaborative process. However, the understanding of how professionals make these contributions and the reasons behind them remains fragmented. Interprofessional collaboration in healthcare requires active contributions from professionals, and it is not solely the responsibility of managers and policymakers. It involves professionals from diverse backgrounds, such as doctors, nurses, data scientists and software engineers, working together to deliver high-quality patient care.

To achieve effective collaboration, professionals need to integrate different perspectives, respect, and trust each other, assume complementary roles, and address the needs of the patients. The active contributions of professionals are crucial in bridging gaps and creating synergy within interprofessional teams.

To facilitate collaboration between healthcare professionals and AI experts, various strategies can be employed. One key strategy is the establishment of interdisciplinary teams and platforms for knowledge sharing. These platforms serve as spaces where professionals from different disciplines can come together, exchange ideas, and collaborate on research and implementation projects. By fostering cross-disciplinary interactions and knowledge sharing, these platforms create opportunities for synergistic collaborations and the integration of diverse perspectives. Regular meetings, workshops, and networking events also play a vital role in promoting collaboration. These gatherings provide opportunities for healthcare professionals and AI experts to engage in face-to-face interactions, build relationships, and share insights. Through these events, professionals can learn from each other, discuss emerging trends, and develop a deeper understanding of each other's expertise. Such interactions can foster cross-pollination of knowledge and ideas, leading to collaborative efforts that drive advancements in AI-driven healthcare. By embracing these strategies for facilitating collaboration and knowledge exchange, healthcare professionals and AI experts can harness the power of teamwork and collective intelligence. Collaborative efforts in AI-driven healthcare have the potential to revolutionize patient care, improve health outcomes, and shape the future of medicine.

Promoting interdisciplinary research and training initiatives in AI and medicine

Interdisciplinary research plays a vital role in advancing healthcare, particularly in the context of AI-driven medicine.

Significance of interdisciplinary research in AI-driven healthcare

Interdisciplinary research offers a unique approach to tackle the multifaceted nature of healthcare challenges and drive innovation in patient care. By bringing together experts from diverse fields, such as medicine, computer science, and data science, interdisciplinary research enables the exploration of uncharted territories and the discovery of novel solutions.[8] One relevant example is the application of remote monitoring in lung transplantation. In a 2012 article from Dimensions in Critical Care Nursing, Arin VanWormer and colleagues, worked together to develop and implement remote monitoring systems to improve patient outcomes and enhance the delivery of person-centered care.[9] By combining expertise from medicine, nursing, and data science, this approach aims to address the challenges associated with post-transplant patient care, such as early detection of complications and real-time monitoring of vital signs.

The framework for this interdisciplinary collaboration is guided by a pulmonary model that integrates the use of telemonitoring and remote monitoring technologies. These technologies allow healthcare professionals to collect and analyze patient data remotely, facilitating continuous monitoring of lung transplant recipients after their procedure. The data collected through remote monitoring can help identify potential issues early on, leading to timely interventions and improved patient care.

By leveraging the expertise of professionals from multiple disciplines, this interdisciplinary research project advanced the use of AI-driven remote monitoring in lung transplantation. It enabled healthcare teams to work collaboratively, share resources and responsibilities, and collectively contribute to enhancing patient outcomes in the field of transplantation. The success of this approach highlights the significance of interdisciplinary research in healthcare, where the combination of diverse perspectives and expertise leads to innovative solutions and improved patient care.

Exploring the potential of interdisciplinary research: Interdisciplinary research has the potential to revolutionize healthcare by leveraging AI technologies. By combining medical expertise with AI-driven tools, researchers can gain new insights into disease prevention, diagnosis, and treatment. For example, deep learning algorithms have shown remarkable capabilities in detecting diabetic retinopathy, classifying skin cancer, and diagnosing cardiac arrhythmias. These advancements highlight the power of interdisciplinary collaboration in improving healthcare outcomes.

Enhancing research outcomes and knowledge discovery: AI technologies, when integrated with interdisciplinary research, offer unprecedented opportunities to enhance research outcomes. AI algorithms can analyze very large amounts of medical data, uncover hidden patterns, and generate valuable insights for personalized medicine. This synergy between AI and interdisciplinary research enables more precise diagnoses, optimized treatment strategies, and improved patient outcomes. By harnessing the potential of AI-driven research, healthcare professionals can navigate complex medical challenges with greater accuracy and efficiency.

Strategies for promoting interdisciplinary research and training

To fully realize the benefits of interdisciplinary research in AI-driven healthcare, it is imperative to foster collaboration and develop a new generation of healthcare professionals equipped with AI skills.

Integrated AI and medicine training programs: Integrated training programs that combine AI and medicine are essential to nurture a new generation of healthcare professionals who possess the necessary interdisciplinary skills.[10] This is not unprecedented, as there are already medical schools, such as Stanford and Harvard, that offer programs that incorporate, research science, law, or business administration degrees with their medical curriculums. These proposed programs should focus on equipping healthcare professionals with AI literacy, data analysis competencies, and an understanding of ethical considerations in AI-driven healthcare. By bridging the gap between AI and medicine, these training programs enable healthcare professionals to harness the potential of AI in their practice.

Showcasing successful collaborations and training initiatives: Highlighting successful examples of interdisciplinary research collaborations and training initiatives can inspire and motivate healthcare professionals to engage in collaborative endeavors. By showcasing real-world cases where interdisciplinary research has positively impacted patient care and healthcare outcomes, professionals gain a deeper understanding of the potential and value of collaboration. These examples can serve as guiding beacons, illustrating the transformative power of interdisciplinary research in healthcare.

Sharing best practices and lessons learned from successful AI implementations in healthcare

Importance of sharing best practices in AI implementations: Sharing successful AI implementation experiences is of paramount importance in driving progress, avoiding pitfalls, and optimizing resource utilization in healthcare. By sharing best practices, healthcare organizations can learn from each other's successes, enabling accelerated advancements in AI adoption. Moreover, sharing both successful and unsuccessful AI implementations fosters continuous learning and improvement within the healthcare community.

To illustrate the potential of AI in healthcare, several case studies can be highlighted. In the field of diagnostics, AI has demonstrated remarkable accuracy in detecting abnormalities in medical images, such as X-rays, MRIs, and CT scans.[11,12] This technology has the potential to enhance diagnostic accuracy, reduce human error, and improve patient outcomes. Additionally, personalized medicine has benefited from AI algorithms that analyze large datasets to tailor treatment plans based on an individual's unique genetic makeup, medical history, and lifestyle factors. AI has also shown promise in patient monitoring, leveraging real-time data from wearable devices and sensors to provide personalized insights and timely interventions.[13]

By sharing experiences, addressing challenges, and implementing recommendations, the healthcare community can maximize the benefits of AI in improving patient care, enhancing clinical decision-making, and advancing medical research.

Conclusion

In the rapidly evolving landscape of AI-driven healthcare, collaboration between healthcare professionals and AI experts is necessary for maximizing the potential of artificial intelligence in advancing patient care, improving decision-making processes, and accelerating innovation. This chapter has explored the critical role of collaborative learning and knowledge sharing in AI-driven healthcare and highlighted strategies for facilitating interdisciplinary research, training initiatives, and sharing best practices in the field.

Collaboration between healthcare professionals and AI experts offers significant benefits for patient care and outcomes. By combining the expertise of healthcare professionals with the analytical capabilities of AI systems, informed decision-making can be enhanced, leading to improved diagnostic accuracy, treatment planning, and predictive modeling. Collaboration also fosters accelerated innovation by enabling the identification of novel solutions and approaches to complex healthcare problems.

However, collaboration between healthcare professionals and AI experts comes with challenges that need to be addressed. Effective communication and understanding between the two groups are essential for successful collaboration. Overcoming communication barriers arising from differences in professional language, perspectives, and knowledge domains is crucial for effective knowledge exchange. Mutual understanding and a shared vision are necessary to align the divergent perspectives of healthcare professionals and AI experts.

To facilitate collaboration and knowledge exchange, various strategies can be employed. Establishing interdisciplinary teams and platforms for knowledge sharing creates spaces where professionals from different disciplines can come together, exchange ideas, and collaborate on research and implementation projects. Regular meetings, workshops, and networking events provide opportunities for face-to-face interactions, relationship building, and insights sharing.

Promoting interdisciplinary research and training initiatives is vital for harnessing the potential of AI-driven healthcare. Integrated AI and medicine training programs equip healthcare professionals with the necessary interdisciplinary skills, AI literacy, data analysis competencies, and ethical considerations. Showcasing successful collaborations and training initiatives inspires and motivates healthcare professionals to engage in collaborative endeavors while sharing best practices enables learning from each other's successes and failures.

Furthermore, sharing experiences and addressing challenges in AI implementation is essential for optimizing its benefits in healthcare. Transparency, ongoing evaluation, and collaboration between multidisciplinary teams are crucial for ensuring the safety, effectiveness, and ethical use of AI systems.

By embracing collaborative learning and knowledge sharing, healthcare professionals and AI experts can collectively shape the future of AI-driven healthcare. Through interdisciplinary research, training initiatives, and the sharing of best practices, the full potential of AI can be harnessed to revolutionize patient care, improve health outcomes, and advance medical research. It is through these collaborative efforts that the transformative power of AI in healthcare can be fully realized.

References

1. Spatharou A, *et al.* (2020) Transforming healthcare with AI: the impact on the workforce and organizations. https://www.mckinsey.com/industries/healthcare/our-insights/transforming-healthcare-with-ai
2. Ahuja AS. (2019) The impact of artificial intelligence in medicine on the future role of the physician. *PeerJ*, **7**, e7702.

3. Bajwa J, Munir U, Nori A, Williams B. (2021) Artificial intelligence in healthcare: transforming the practice of medicine. *Future Healthcare Journal*, **8**(2), e188–e194.

4. Haupt CE, Marks M. (2023) AI-generated medical advice-GPT and beyond. *JAMA Network*, **329**, 1349.

5. Hannun AY, Rajpurkar P, Haghpanahi M, Tison GH, Bourn C, Turakhia MP, Ng AY. (2019) Cardiologist-level arrhythmia detection and classification in ambulatory electrocardiograms using a deep neural network. *Nature Medicine*, **25**(1), 65–69. Erratum in: *Nature Medicine*, **25**(3), 530.

6. González-Gonzalo C, *et al.* (2022) Trustworthy AI: closing the gap between development and integration of AI systems in ophthalmic practice. *Progress in Retinal and Eye Research*, **90**(September), 101034.

7. Schot E, Tummers L, Noordegraaf M. Working on working together. A systematic review on how healthcare professionals contribute to interprofessional collaboration. *J Interprof Care*. 2020 May–Jun, **34**(3), 332–342. doi: 10.1080/13561820.2019.1636007. Epub 2019 Jul 22. PMID: 31329469.

8. Ledford H. (2015) How to solve the world's biggest problems. *Nature*, **525**, 308–311.

9. VanWormer A, Lindquist R, Robiner W, Finkelstein S. Interdisciplinary collaboration applied to clinical research: an example of remote monitoring in lung transplantation. *Dimens Crit Care Nurs*. 2012 May–Jun, **31**(3), 202–10. doi: 10.1097/DCC.0b013e31824e0307. PMID: 22475710; PMCID: PMC3320716.

10. Topol, Eric. Deep medicine: how artificial intelligence can make healthcare human again. Basic Books, 2019. pages 186–187.

11. Hosny A, Parmar C, Quackenbush J, Schwartz LH, Aerts HJWL. Artificial intelligence in radiology. *Nat Rev Cancer*. 2018 Aug, **18**(8), 500–510. doi: 10.1038/s41568-018-0016-5. PMID: 29777175; PMCID: PMC6268174.

12. Jin D, Harrison AP, Zhang L, Yan K, Wang Y, Cai J, Miao S, Lu L. Artificial intelligence in radiology. *Artificial Intelligence in Medicine*. 2021 265–89. doi: 10.1016/B978-0-12-821259-2.00014-4. Epub 2020 Sep 11. PMCID: PMC7484814.

13. Shaik T, Tao X, Higgins N, *et al*, Remote patient monitoring using artificial intelligence: Current state, applications, and challenges, Wires Volume13, Issue2, March/April 2023, e1485.

Chapter 18

Future Trends and Emerging Technologies in AI-Driven Healthcare

Introduction

The healthcare landscape is undergoing a rapid transformation, fueled by the remarkable progress of artificial intelligence (AI) and its potential to revolutionize patient care and medical practices. As AI continues to advance, it opens new horizons for healthcare professionals, researchers, and technologists to explore and harness its transformative power. Understanding the future trends and emerging technologies in AI-driven healthcare is of utmost importance to unlock its full potential and shape the future of medicine.

This chapter delves into the exciting realm of AI-driven healthcare, providing insights into the latest advancements and trends that are reshaping the industry. By exploring the future directions and emerging technologies in this field, this chapter aims to equip healthcare professionals, researchers, and AI experts with the knowledge necessary to navigate this evolving landscape and embrace the transformative potential of AI in patient care. Throughout this chapter, we will look into five key areas that are at the forefront of AI-driven healthcare innovation. We will start by exploring AI in diagnostics and imaging, where AI algorithms and deep learning (DL) techniques are revolutionizing medical image analysis, enabling automated disease detection, and enhancing diagnostic accuracy. Then, moving on to AI-assisted surgery and robotics, where AI technologies are revolutionizing surgical procedures, providing surgeons with enhanced precision, visualization, and control, leading to improved patient outcomes. Followed by AI-enabled patient monitoring and personalized care, where wearable devices, remote monitoring, and AI algorithms converge to continuously monitor patients, predict disease progression, assess risks, and develop personalized treatment plans. Next, we will explore AI in drug discovery and precision medicine, where AI plays a pivotal role in accelerating drug discovery, enabling personalized medicine approaches, and revolutionizing the development of therapeutics. Lastly, AI-driven healthcare operations and resource management will be discussed, focusing on the optimization of resource allocation, scheduling, and patient flow through the application of AI-powered solutions. We will examine how predictive analytics and machine learning algorithms can enhance decision support systems, enabling efficient staffing, inventory management, and equipment maintenance.

By venturing into these key areas, we hope to provide a comprehensive overview of the future trends and emerging technologies in AI-driven healthcare. This chapter will address the potential benefits, challenges, and ethical considerations associated with the integration of AI in healthcare. Through responsible implementation and continuous research, AI has the potential to significantly improve patient outcomes, optimize resource utilization, and shape the future of medicine.

AI in diagnostics and imaging

Medical imaging plays a pivotal role in diagnosing and monitoring diseases, guiding treatment decisions, and assessing treatment effectiveness. The integration of AI algorithms and DL techniques has brought about a paradigm shift in diagnostic imaging, empowering healthcare professionals with enhanced accuracy, efficiency, and novel insights. This section will explore the future trends and emerging technologies in AI-driven diagnostics and imaging, highlighting their transformative potential in revolutionizing healthcare outcomes. Utilizing AI algorithms and DL techniques, AI-driven diagnostics and imaging have made significant strides in enhancing accuracy and efficiency. The ability of AI models to learn from enormous amounts of data and identify complex patterns has enabled breakthroughs in medical image analysis. AI algorithms can now automatically detect and classify diseases with remarkable precision, reducing the reliance on manual interpretation and enhancing diagnostic capabilities. By leveraging DL techniques, AI can extract intricate features from medical images, enabling the detection of subtle abnormalities that may be challenging for human observers to identify.

Radiology and pathology are two areas where the integration of AI has shown tremendous promise. In radiology, AI algorithms can assist radiologists in interpreting medical images, aiding in the identification of anomalies, such as tumors, fractures, and lesions, with greater accuracy. AI-powered systems can quickly analyze large volumes of imaging data, providing radiologists with valuable insights for diagnosis and treatment planning. Additionally, AI algorithms can speed up radiology report generation, leading to faster turnaround times and improved workflow efficiency. In pathology, AI has the potential to revolutionize the field by augmenting the capabilities of pathologists. AI algorithms can analyze digital pathology images, aiding in the detection and classification of cancerous cells, improving diagnostic accuracy, and enabling more personalized treatment strategies.[1,2] One study showed that by using AI, pathologists have decreased their error rate in recognizing cancer-positive lymph nodes from 3.4% to 0.5%.[3] By leveraging AI in pathology, healthcare providers can enhance patient care by facilitating timely and precise diagnoses. As an example, the presence of lymph node (LN) metastasis is one of the most important prognostic factors in determining cancer stage and guiding treatment decisions.[4] However, manually screening lymph nodes for metastatic tumor cells is labor intensive and susceptible to error. Many hospitals also require rapid intraoperative sentinel lymph node analysis to guide surgery,[5] further increasing the workload of pathologists. Currently, pathologists may need to meticulously examine numerous conventional H&E and IHC-stained slides to detect micrometastases and isolated tumor cells. Automated AI analysis of lymph node histopathology slides could improve detection of LN metastases that impact staging and treatment, while reducing the workload of pathologists. By digitizing whole slide images, AI and DL algorithms can rapidly analyze the histopathology of the slides.[6] This technology has the potential to ease the workload of pathologists and increase diagnostic accuracy.[7]

Looking ahead, the future of AI in diagnostics and imaging holds immense promise. AI has the potential to transform early disease detection and prevention, leading to improved healthcare outcomes. By analyzing large datasets and integrating various clinical and non-clinical data sources, AI algorithms can identify subtle biomarkers and risk factors that may indicate the presence of a disease even before symptoms manifest. This early detection and intervention can significantly improve patient prognosis and survival rates. Moreover, AI-driven diagnostics and imaging are evolving to embrace multimodal approaches.[8] Integrating multiple imaging modalities, such as magnetic resonance imaging (MRI), computed tomography (CT), and positron emission tomography (PET), with AI algorithms can provide a comprehensive view of diseases, enabling more accurate and holistic diagnoses.[9,10] This multimodal integration, combined with AI-driven analysis, has the potential to unlock new insights into disease progression, treatment response, and personalized medicine approaches.

AI-assisted surgery and robotics

Surgical procedures are complex and demanding, requiring precision, expertise, and utmost care. The integration of AI technologies in surgery has opened new possibilities for improving surgical outcomes and enhancing patient care. This section examines the applications of AI in surgical procedures, focusing on robotic-assisted surgeries and virtual reality simulations, investigates how AI can enhance precision, visualization, and control in surgical interventions, and discusses real-world examples that demonstrate the potential benefits of AI-driven surgical systems. Additionally, the ethical considerations and challenges associated with implementing AI in surgical settings will be addressed.

Applications of AI in surgical procedures

The integration of AI in surgery, particularly in robotic-assisted surgeries and virtual reality simulations, holds immense potential for improving surgical outcomes and patient care.

Human surgeons must manage physical, mental, and technical factors during surgery that impact outcomes. Fatigue, tremors, and lapses in concentration can negatively affect surgical performance. Robotic surgical systems aim to provide advantages over human limitations that lead to variability. For instance, robots do not experience fatigue or tremors, have motion scaling for precision, and a wider range of axial movement. In the future, advancements in surgical AI could optimize robots, consistently assisting human surgeons by addressing variations in individual performance. AI technologies enable enhanced precision, visualization, and control during surgical interventions, leading to reduced invasiveness and improved patient outcomes. Real-world examples, such as the da Vinci Surgical System and the ROSA robotic surgical assistant, showcase the transformative impact of AI in surgical practices.

Robotic-assisted surgeries

These robotic systems can be used in various surgical domains, including urology, gynecology, cardiac surgery, and orthopedics. For example, the da Vinci Surgical System enables surgeons to perform minimally invasive procedures with greater accuracy and less tissue damage and blood loss.[11] By leveraging AI algorithms, these robotic systems can enhance surgical capabilities and overcome the limitations of traditional surgical techniques.

Virtual reality simulations

Virtual reality (VR) simulations have emerged as a valuable tool in surgical training and preoperative planning.[12] AI-driven VR simulations provide surgeons with realistic environments to practice complex procedures and improve their skills. Surgeons can perform virtual surgeries on patient-specific anatomical models, enabling them to develop proficiency and explore different surgical approaches. These simulations also allow surgeons to anticipate potential challenges and optimize surgical plans, leading to improved patient outcomes.

Enhanced precision, visualization, and control

AI technologies offer several benefits in terms of precision, visualization, and control during surgical interventions. By integrating AI algorithms, surgical systems can analyze real-time data, such as images and sensor inputs, to provide surgeons with enhanced information and guidance.[14] For instance, AI-powered image analysis can assist surgeons in identifying critical structures, navigating complex anatomies, and detecting subtle abnormalities.[15] Additionally, AI algorithms can analyze intraoperative data to provide feedback and optimize surgical workflows, leading to more precise and efficient procedures. For instance, an AI system was able to analyze real-time laparoscopic video during sleeve gastrectomy procedures and identify the surgical steps with 92.8% accuracy, while also detecting any missing or unexpected steps.[16] The ROSA robotic surgical assistant system is utilized in neurosurgery to enhance precision and control during delicate procedures. By leveraging AI algorithms and robotic arms, ROSA assists surgeons in accurately placing electrodes for deep brain stimulation, improving outcomes for patients with movement disorders like Parkinson's disease.[17]

Potential benefits of AI-driven surgical systems

AI-driven surgical systems offer numerous potential benefits that can positively impact patient outcomes and healthcare practices. One of the benefits include reduced invasiveness. For example, AI technologies, particularly robotic-assisted surgeries, can enable minimally invasive procedures. This approach results in smaller incisions, reduced pain, shorter hospital stays, and faster recovery times for patients. By enhancing precision, visualization, and control, AI-driven surgical systems have the potential to improve surgical outcomes. Surgeons can perform complex procedures with greater accuracy, leading to reduced complications, improved functional outcomes, and increased patient satisfaction. The use of the da Vinci Surgical System in prostate cancer surgeries has shown promising outcomes. The system's AI-powered robotic arms enable surgeons to perform precise, nerve-sparing procedures, resulting in improved urinary continence and sexual function outcomes for patients.[18]

AI-enabled patient monitoring and personalized care

Advancements in AI have paved the way for innovative approaches to patient monitoring and personalized care. This section explores the utilization of wearable devices, remote monitoring, and AI algorithms for continuous patient monitoring, the development of AI-driven prediction models for disease progression and risk assessment, and the empowerment of patients through improved engagement and self-management using AI-powered mobile applications and virtual assistants.

Harnessing the power of wearable devices, remote monitoring, and AI algorithms

Wearable devices

AI-enabled wearable devices, such as smartwatches and fitness trackers, provide healthcare professionals with real-time data on patients' vital signs, activity levels, and sleep patterns.[19] These devices can track indicators of various health conditions and detect anomalies, enabling early intervention and timely medical attention. An example of this is the use of AI-powered wearable ECG monitors, which allow patients with cardiac conditions to continuously monitor their heart rhythm and receive alerts in case of abnormalities, empowering both patients and healthcare providers to detect potential cardiac events.[20]

Remote monitoring

AI facilitates remote monitoring by analyzing patient-generated data transmitted from home devices, such as blood pressure monitors or glucose meters. This approach allows healthcare professionals to remotely monitor patients' health status, identify trends, and intervene promptly when necessary. Remote monitoring increases the quality of medical care because it lowers the chance of further complications and hospital admission.[21] One example of this is AI algorithms integrated into remote glucose monitoring systems, which can analyze blood sugar trends and patterns, providing personalized insights to diabetes patients and their healthcare providers for better glycemic control.[22]

Developing AI-driven prediction models for disease progression and risk assessment

Disease progression

AI algorithms can analyze patient data, including medical records and imaging results, to predict disease progression. By identifying early signs of deterioration or progression, healthcare professionals can intervene with timely interventions and personalized treatment plans. For example, AI algorithms applied to longitudinal data of multiple sclerosis patients can predict disease progression and help tailor treatment strategies accordingly, improving outcomes and quality of life for these patients.[23,24]

Risk assessment

AI-driven prediction models can assess patients' risk of developing certain conditions, such as cardiovascular diseases or cancer, based on a combination of clinical data, genetic markers, and lifestyle factors. This allows for targeted preventive measures and interventions. AI-based risk assessment tools in cardiovascular medicine can evaluate patient data, including demographics, medical history, and lab results, to predict the likelihood of future cardiovascular events, enabling personalized prevention strategies.[25] Similarly, machine learning algorithms can classify cancer patients into high or low risk groups and improve our understanding of cancer progression.[26]

Empowering patients through improved engagement and self-management

AI-powered mobile applications

Mobile applications utilizing AI algorithms can provide patients with personalized health recommendations, medication reminders, and access to educational resources.[27] These apps enhance patient engagement and promote self-management of their health conditions.[28] AI-powered mobile applications for asthma management can provide real-time air quality data, personalized triggers identification, and medication reminders, empowering patients to effectively manage their condition and reduce the frequency of asthma attacks.[29]

Virtual assistants

AI-driven virtual assistants, such as voice-activated devices or chatbots, offer patients access to personalized healthcare information, appointment scheduling, and medication management.[30] These virtual assistants provide convenient and timely support to patients, enhancing their overall healthcare experience. Voice-activated virtual assistants can help patients with chronic conditions, such as diabetes, by answering questions, providing lifestyle recommendations, assisting with medication adherence, promoting self-care and patient empowerment.[31,32]

In conclusion, the integration of AI in patient monitoring and personalized care holds significant promise for improving healthcare outcomes and empowering patients to actively participate in their care. Through the utilization of wearable devices, remote monitoring, AI prediction models, and AI-powered applications, healthcare professionals can access valuable insights, deliver personalized interventions, and enhance patient engagement. However, it is crucial to address ethical considerations, including patient privacy, data security, and responsible AI use to ensure patient trust and the ethical implementation of these technologies in healthcare practice. By striking a balance between technological advancements and patient-centric care, healthcare professionals can leverage the potential of AI to revolutionize patient monitoring and personalized care.

AI in drug discovery and precision medicine

In recent years, the intersection of AI and healthcare has shown immense promise in revolutionizing drug discovery and precision medicine.[33] The integration of AI with precision medicine techniques has the power to transform healthcare. On one hand, precision medicine identifies specific phenotypes and biological factors that affect how patients respond to treatment, targeting care to individual needs. On the other hand, AI provides the advanced analytical capabilities to spot new patterns and derive insights from the wealth of patient data. Together, AI and precision medicine can enable truly personalized diagnoses and prognoses by holistically assessing each person's unique genomic makeup, health history, symptoms, and lifestyle. AI models can continuously learn from new data to refine predictions and recommendations tailored to each patient. This augmented intelligence supports clinicians in providing the optimal care for the specific patient at the appropriate time. Ongoing research on combining precision medicine datasets with AI will likely solve some of healthcare's greatest challenges, propelling us toward accurate, individualized treatment plans. By leveraging AI-driven technologies, healthcare professionals are exploring innovative approaches to accelerate the discovery of new drugs, identify potential therapeutic targets, and personalize treatment strategies.

Accelerating drug discovery

AI plays a crucial role in expediting the drug discovery process by streamlining various stages, from target identification to virtual screening of potential therapeutics.[34] With the ability to analyze huge amounts of data, AI algorithms can identify patterns, predict molecular interactions, and propose novel drug candidates. Several companies are actively utilizing AI technology to accelerate drug discovery and target identification. Here are just a few examples:

- BenevolentAI: BenevolentAI is a leading AI-driven drug discovery company that employs machine learning algorithms to analyze large amounts of biomedical data, including scientific literature, clinical trial data, and molecular databases.[35] Their AI platform helps identify novel drug targets, predict drug interactions, and prioritize potential therapeutic candidates for further investigation.
- Insilico Medicine: Insilico Medicine utilizes AI and deep learning algorithms to expedite the drug discovery process.[36] Their AI-driven

platform analyzes large datasets, such as genomic data and molecular structures, to predict the efficacy and safety of potential drug candidates. They also employ generative adversarial networks (GANs) to generate novel drug-like molecules for specific targets.

- Atomwise: Atomwise harnesses the power of AI for virtual screening and drug discovery.[37] Their AI platform employs deep learning algorithms to analyze molecular structures and predict the binding affinity of small molecules to specific targets. This enables rapid identification of potential drug candidates, thus, reducing the time and cost associated with traditional screening methods.
- BPGbio: BPGbio integrates AI and systems biology to accelerate the discovery of new drugs. Their AI-driven platform analyzes multiomic data, including genomics, proteomics, and metabolomics, to uncover novel therapeutic targets and identify potential drug candidates. They also utilize AI algorithms to predict drug efficacy and personalize treatment approaches.
- Cyclica: Cyclica combines AI and computational biophysics to accelerate the drug discovery process.[39] Their AI platform, Ligand Express, analyzes large molecular databases to predict drug-target interactions, assess target druggability, and prioritize potential therapeutic compounds. This approach facilitates the identification of novel drug candidates and enhances target identification.

Other examples include AI algorithms that analyze large molecular databases, predict drug-target interactions, and prioritize potential drug candidates for further investigation. These AI techniques enable healthcare professionals to make informed decisions regarding which compounds to pursue, thereby reducing the time and resources required for traditional trial-and-error approaches.

Personalized medicine approaches

AI-driven analysis of genomic and clinical data has opened new avenues for personalized medicine. By integrating patient-specific information with AI algorithms, healthcare professionals can tailor treatment plans to individual patients, considering their genetic makeup, disease characteristics, and other relevant factors.[33] AI helps identify biomarkers associated with specific diseases, predict treatment responses, and guide the selection of optimal therapies. This approach enhances patient outcomes by optimizing treatment efficacy while minimizing adverse reactions.

Examples include AI algorithms that analyze genomics data to identify mutations associated with drug response and predict patient-specific treatment outcomes. An example of a company that uses AI to provide precision health is Tempus Health.[40] Tempus Health harnesses the power of AI to analyze genomic data and identify genetic variations that contribute to disease development and progression. Through advanced machine learning algorithms, the company can detect subtle genetic patterns associated with specific conditions, allowing for early detection and targeted interventions. By examining the DNA sequences and variations within a patient's genome, Tempus Health can identify potential genetic drivers of diseases, enabling healthcare professionals to develop precise treatment strategies and recommend appropriate therapies or clinical trials tailored to individual patients.

Prediction of treatment response and adverse reactions

AI enables the prediction of treatment response and adverse reactions by leveraging machine learning models trained on diverse patient data.[41] By analyzing factors such as patient demographics, disease characteristics, genetic variations, and treatment history, AI algorithms can identify patterns that correlate with treatment outcomes. This empowers healthcare professionals to predict the effectiveness of specific treatments for individual patients, optimize treatment plans, anticipate potential adverse reactions, and monitor patients more effectively. AI algorithms can also assist in identifying optimal drug combinations for synergistic effects, maximizing treatment efficacy. Examples of this include AI models that predict the response to cancer therapies based on molecular profiles of tumors and clinical data.[42,43]

Impact on cost and time

The integration of AI in drug discovery and precision medicine has the potential to significantly reduce costs and timelines associated with traditional drug development. By leveraging AI for virtual screening and prioritization of drug candidates, researchers can focus resources on the most promising candidates, thereby reducing the costs associated with unsuccessful drug development.[44] Additionally, AI-enabled predictive models can optimize clinical trial design, patient selection, and dosage determination, further enhancing efficiency and cost-effectiveness.[45] Examples include AI algorithms that expedite the identification of potential drug targets and reduce the time and resources required for preclinical and clinical testing.[46,47]

In conclusion, AI-driven approaches in drug discovery and precision medicine hold immense potential to transform healthcare practices. By leveraging AI technologies, healthcare professionals can accelerate the discovery of new drugs, personalize treatment strategies, predict treatment outcomes, and optimize drug combinations. These advancements not only improve patient outcomes but also have the potential to reduce costs and timelines associated with drug development. As the development of AI continues, it will play an increasingly vital role in shaping the future of drug discovery and precision medicine.

AI-driven healthcare operations and resource management

AI has emerged as a powerful tool for optimizing healthcare operations and resource management, enabling healthcare professionals to enhance efficiency, streamline workflows, and improve patient outcomes. By leveraging predictive analytics, machine learning algorithms, and decision support systems, AI-driven solutions can revolutionize resource allocation, scheduling, and patient flow within healthcare facilities.[48,49]

One notable application of AI in healthcare operations is in optimizing resource allocation and scheduling. AI algorithms can analyze historical data, patient demographics, and clinical information to forecast patient demand and allocate resources accordingly. For example, AI-powered systems can predict patient admissions, emergency department visits, and surgical caseloads, allowing healthcare professionals to allocate staff, beds, and operating rooms efficiently.[50] This enables healthcare facilities to optimize resource utilization, reduce wait times, and improve patient access to care.

Moreover, AI-driven predictive analytics can assist in inventory management and supply chain optimization.[51] By analyzing historical data, consumption patterns, and patient needs, AI algorithms can predict demand for medications, medical supplies, and equipment. This enables healthcare professionals to maintain optimal inventory levels, reduce wastage, and ensure timely availability of critical resources. For instance, AI systems can forecast medication demand based on patient diagnoses, prescription patterns, and disease outbreaks, facilitating proactive inventory management.[52]

AI also plays a crucial role in enhancing decision support systems for staffing and workforce management. Recent studies have indicated that the persistent staffing shortages in healthcare will likely lead to extended patient wait times as well as a significant decline in the overall quality of medical care provided.[53–55]

The stochasticity of clinical operations, such as patient discharges and arrivals, diagnostic tests needed, and durations of treatment impose challenges to predict future demands on staffing and materials on managers. By analyzing factors such as patient acuity, staff availability, and skill sets, AI algorithms can generate optimized staffing schedules.[56,57] These schedules consider patient needs, workload distribution, and staff preferences, ensuring adequate coverage and improved workflow efficiency. AI-powered systems can also facilitate real-time monitoring of staff performance and workload, enabling healthcare professionals to make informed decisions regarding staffing adjustments. This can lead to increased healthcare worker productivity. For example, in nursing, the use of AI-enabled tools has increased productivity by 30% to 50%.[58]

These are some examples of AI-driven healthcare operations and resource management solutions:

- GE Healthcare's Capacity Command Center[59]: This AI-powered system leverages predictive analytics and real-time data to optimize patient flow, bed allocation, and staff assignments within hospitals. By analyzing historical and real-time data, the system provides actionable insights to healthcare professionals, enabling them to proactively manage patient demand and optimize resource utilization.

- Qventus[60]: Qventus offers an AI-based operations management platform that assists healthcare professionals in optimizing workflows, reducing patient wait times, and improving operational efficiency. The platform leverages machine learning algorithms to predict patient demand, identify bottlenecks, and generate real-time recommendations for resource allocation and scheduling.
- Cerner's Command Center[61]: Cerner's AI-driven Command Center solution integrates real-time data from various healthcare systems to provide healthcare professionals with comprehensive insights for operational decision-making. The platform uses predictive analytics to forecast patient flow, optimize bed utilization, and support efficient resource allocation.

These examples highlight how AI-driven solutions can empower healthcare professionals to optimize healthcare operations, allocate resources effectively, and enhance patient care delivery. By embracing AI technology, healthcare professionals can streamline workflows, improve resource utilization, and ultimately provide more efficient and patient-centric care.

Conclusion

As we look towards the future, the integration of AI in healthcare continues to hold immense potential for transformative advancements. The convergence of cutting-edge technologies such as deep learning, natural language processing, and robotics offers exciting possibilities for improving medical diagnostics, treatment strategies, and patient outcomes. The impact of AI on personalized medicine and precision healthcare is expected to increase, allowing for tailored interventions and predictive models that enhance patient care. As we consider the potential impact of AI on the future of medicine, it is essential to embrace ongoing research and nurture collaborations between healthcare professionals and AI experts. By fostering interdisciplinary partnerships, we can further explore the frontiers of AI in medicine, opening new avenues for innovation and ultimately improving the delivery of healthcare worldwide. With a continued focus on ethics, transparency, and patient-centered care, AI has the potential to revolutionize the medical field, ushering in an era of enhanced diagnostics, optimized treatments, and improved patient outcomes.

References

1. Liu Y, Kohlberger T, Norouzi M, Dahl GE, Smith JL, Mohtashamian A, Olson N, Peng LH, Hipp JD, Stumpe MC. (2019) Artificial intelligence-based breast cancer nodal metastasis detection: insights into the black box for pathologists. *Archives of Pathology & Laboratory Medicine*, **143**(7), 859–868.
2. Caldonazzi N, Rizzo PC, Eccher A, Girolami I, Fanelli GN, Naccarato AG, Bonizzi G, Fusco N, d'Amati G, Scarpa A, Pantanowitz L, Marletta S. (2023) Value of artificial intelligence in evaluating lymph node metastases. *Cancers (Basel)*, **15**(9), 2491.
3. Ting Sim JZ, Fong QW, Huang W, Tan CH. (2023) Machine learning in medicine: What clinicians should know. *Singapore Medical Journal*, **64**(2), 91–97.
4. Amin MB, *et al.* (2017) *AJCC Cancer Staging Manual, 8th edition.* Springer; Berlin/Heidelberg, Germany: American Joint Commission on Cancer, Chicago, IL, USA.
5. Girolami I, Neri S, Eccher A, Brunelli M, Hanna M, Pantanowitz L, Hanspeter E, Mazzoleni G. (2022) Frozen section telepathology service: efficiency and benefits of an e-health policy in South Tyrol. *Digital Health*, **8**, 20552076221116776.
6. Tizhoosh HR, Pantanowitz L. (2018) artificial intelligence and digital pathology: challenges and opportunities. *Journal of Pathology Informatics*, **9**, 38.
7. Caldonazzi N, Rizzo PC, Eccher A, Girolami I, Fanelli GN, Naccarato AG, Bonizzi G, Fusco N, d'Amati G, Scarpa A, Pantanowitz L, Marletta S. (2023) Value of artificial intelligence in evaluating lymph node metastases. *Cancers*, **15**(9), 2491.
8. Maragna R, Giacari C, Guglielmo M, *et al.* (2021) Artificial intelligence based multimodality imaging: a new frontier in coronary artery disease management. *Frontiers in Cardiovascular Medicine*, **8**, 736223.
9. Litjens G, Kooi T, Bejnordi BE, Setio AAA, Ciompi F, Ghafoorian M, van der Laak JAWM, van Ginneken B, Sánchez CI. (2017) A survey on deep learning in medical image analysis. *Medical Image Analysis*, **42**, 60–88.

10. Huang SC, Pareek A, Zamanian R, Banerjee I, Lungren MP. (2020) Multimodal fusion with deep neural networks for leveraging CT imaging and electronic health record: a case-study in pulmonary embolism detection. *Scientific Reports*, **10**(1), 22147.
11. Weber PA, Merola S, Wasielewski A, Ballantyne GH. (2002) Telerobotic-assisted laparoscopic right and sigmoid colectomies for benign disease. *Diseases of the Colon & Rectum*, **45**, 1689–1694.
12. Shah J, Vyas A, Vyas D. (2014) The history of robotics in surgical specialties. *American Journal of Robotic Surgery*, **1**(1), 12–20.
13. Lan L, Mao RQ, Qiu RY, Kay J, de Sa D. (2023) Immersive virtual reality for patient-specific preoperative planning: a systematic review. *Surgical Innovation*, **30**(1), 109–122.
14. Tang R, Yang W, Hou Y, Yu L, Wu G, Tong X, Yan J, Lu Q. (2021) Augmented reality-assisted pancreaticoduodenectomy with superior mesenteric vein resection and reconstruction. *Gastroenterology Research and Practice*, **2021**, 9621323.
15. Ali S. (2022) Where do we stand in AI for endoscopic image analysis? Deciphering gaps and future directions. *npj Digital Medicine*, **5**, 184 (2022).
16. Volkov M, Hashimoto DA, Rosman G, *et al.* (2017) Machine learning and coresets for automated real-time video segmentation of laparoscopic and robot-assisted surgery. *IEEE International Conference on Robotics and Automation*, 754–759.
17. Faraji AH, Kokkinos V, Sweat JC, Crammond DJ, Richardson RM. (2020) Robotic-Assisted Stereotaxy for deep brain stimulation lead implantation in awake patients. *Operative neurosurgery (Hagerstown)*, **19**(4), 444–452.
18. Yaxley JW, Coughlin GD, Chambers SK, Occhipinti S, Samaratunga H, Zajdlewicz L, Dunglison N, Carter R, Williams S, Payton DJ, Perry-Keene J, Lavin MF, Gardiner RA. (2016) Robot-assisted laparoscopic prostatectomy versus open radical retropubic prostatectomy: early outcomes from a randomised controlled phase 3 study. *The Lancet*, **388**(10049), 1057–1066. Erratum in: **389**(10077), e5.
19. Sabry F, Eltaras T, Labda W, Alzoubi K, Malluhi Q. (2022) Machine learning for healthcare wearable devices: the big picture. *Journal of Healthcare Engineering*, **2022**, 4653923.
20. Neri L, Oberdier MT, van Abeelen KCJ, Menghini L, Tumarkin E, Tripathi H, Jaipalli S, Orro A, Paolocci N, Gallelli I, Dall'Olio M, Beker A, Carrick RT, Borghi C, Halperin HR. (2023) Electrocardiogram monitoring wearable devices and artificial-intelligence-enabled diagnostic capabilities: a review. *Sensors*, **23**(10), 4805.

21. Lu JW, Wang Y, Sun Y, *et al.* (2021) Effectiveness of telemonitoring for reducing exacerbation occurrence in COPD patients with past exacerbation history: a systematic review and meta-analysis. *Frontiers in Medicine*, **8**, 720019.

22. Vettoretti M, Cappon G, Facchinetti A, Sparacino G. (2020) Advanced diabetes management using artificial intelligence and continuous glucose monitoring sensors. *Sensors*, **20**(14), 3870.

23. Bonacchi R, Filippi M, Rocca MA. (2022) Role of artificial intelligence in MS clinical practice. *NeuroImage: Clinical*, **35**, 103065.

24. De Brouwer E, *et al.* (2021) Longitudinal machine learning modeling of MS patient trajectories improves predictions of disability progression. *Computer Methods and Programs in Biomedicine*, **208**(September), 106180.

25. Weng SF, Reps J, Kai J, Garibaldi JM, Qureshi N. (2017) Can machine-learning improve cardiovascular risk prediction using routine clinical data? PLOS One, **12**(4), e0174944.

26. Kourou K, Exarchos TP, Exarchos KP, Karamouzis MV, Fotiadis DI. (2014) Machine learning applications in cancer prognosis and prediction. *Computational and Structural Biotechnology Journal*, **13**, 8–17.

27. Babel A, Taneja R, Mondello Malvestiti F, Monaco A, Donde S. (2021) Artificial intelligence solutions to increase medication adherence in patients with non-communicable diseases. *Frontiers in Digital Health*, **3**, 669869.

28. AITJ Staff Writer. (2023) Fostering patient engagement: how mobile apps revolutionize healthcare software development. https://www.aitimejournal. com/fostering-patient-engagement-how-mobile-apps-revolutionize-health-care-software-development/45833/#:~:text=Moreover%2C%20mobile%20 healthcare%20applications%20can,outcomes%20and%20more%20effec-tive%20treatments

29. (2023) CMI Health rolls out new app-based asthma-management platform. https://www.medicaldevice-network.com/news/cmi-health-rasthma-management-platform/

30. Xu L, Sanders L, Li K, Chow JCL. (2021) Chatbot for health care and oncology applications using artificial intelligence and machine learning: systematic review. *JMIR Cancer*, **7**(4), e27850.

31. Patel MS, Asch DA, Volpp KG. (2015) Wearable devices as facilitators, not drivers, of health behavior change. *JAMA Network*, **313**(5), 459–460.

32. Jadczyk T, Wojakowski W, Tendera M, Henry TD, Egnaczyk G, Shreenivas S. (2021) Artificial intelligence can improve patient management at the time of a pandemic: the role of voice technology. *Journal of Medical Internet Research*, **23**(5), e22959.

33. Johnson KB, Wei WQ, Weeraratne D, Frisse ME, Misulis K, Rhee K, Zhao J, Snowdon JL. (2021) Precision medicine, AI, and the future of personalized health care. *Clinical and Translational Science*, **14**(1), 86–93.

34. Blanco-González A, Cabezón A, Seco-González A, Conde-Torres D, Antelo-Riveiro P, Piñeiro Á, Garcia-Fandino R. (2023) The role of AI in drug discovery: challenges, opportunities, and strategies. *Pharmaceuticals*, **16**(6), 891.

35. Complex biology, unlocked. https://www.benevolent.com/

36. Artificial intelligence for every step of pharmaceutical research and development. https://insilico.com/

37. Artificial intelligence for drug discovery. https://www.atomwise.com/

38. Transforming drug discovery with artificial intelligence. https://bpgbio.com/

39. From molecule to medicine. https://cyclicarx.com/

40. AI-enabled precision medicine. https://www.tempus.com/

41. Sheu Yh, Magdamo C, Miller M, *et al.* (2023) AI-assisted prediction of differential response to antidepressant classes using electronic health records. *npj Digital Medicine*, **6**, 73. https://doi.org/10.1038/s41746-023-00817-8

42. Bhinder B, Gilvary C, Madhukar NS, Elemento O. (2021) Artificial intelligence in cancer research and precision medicine. *Cancer Discovery*, **11**(4), 900–915.

43. Huang C, Clayton EA, Matyunina LV, *et al.* (2018) Machine learning predicts individual cancer patient responses to therapeutic drugs with high accuracy. *Scientific Reports*, **8**, 16444.

44. Vijayan RSK, Kihlberg J, Cross JB, Poongavanam V. (2022) Enhancing preclinical drug discovery with artificial intelligence. *Drug Discovery Today*, **27**(4), 967–984.

45. Cascini F, Beccia F, Causio FA, Melnyk A, Zaino A, Ricciardi W. (2022) Scoping review of the current landscape of AI-based applications in clinical trials. *Frontiers in Public Health*, **10**, 949377. doi: 10.3389/fpubh.2022. 949377. PMID: 36033816; PMCID: PMC9414344.

46. Duch W. (2007) Artificial intelligence approaches for rational drug design and discovery. *Current Pharmaceutical Design*, **13**, 1497–1508.

47. Mak K-K, Pichika MR. (2019) Artificial intelligence in drug development: present status and future prospects. *Drug Discovery Today*, **24**, 773–780.

48. Dawoodbhoy FM, Delaney J, Cecula P, Yu J, Peacock I, Tan J, Cox B. (2021) AI in patient flow: applications of artificial intelligence to improve patient flow in NHS acute mental health inpatient units. *Heliyon*, **7**(5), e06993.

49. How AI can take optimised healthcare resource utilisation to the next level. (2021) https://www.healthcareitnews.com/news/asia/how-ai-can-take-optimised-healthcare-resource-utilisation-next-level

50. Nguyen D, Fu B, Zhou M, Soriano A, Sun Z, Burattin A. (2021) Predicting patientcare demand in hospital emergency departments using machine learning and routing simulations. *Expert Systems with Applications*, **184**, 115487.

51. Zamani ED, Smyth C, Gupta S, Dennehy D. (2022) Artificial intelligence and big data analytics for supply chain resilience: a systematic literature review. *Annals of Operations Research*, **30**, 1–28.

52. Khan O, Parvez M, Kumari P, Parvez S, Ahmad S. (2023) The future of pharmacy: how AI is revolutionizing the industry. *Intelligent Pharmacy*, **1**(1), 32–40.

53. Hassmiller SB, Cozine M. (2006) Addressing the nurse shortage to improve the quality of patient care. *Health Affairs (Millwood)*. **25**(1), 268–274.

54. Dall T, West T, Chakrabarti R, Reynolds R, Iacobucci W. (2018) *2018 update. The complexities of physician supply and demand: projections from 2016 to 2030*. Washington, DC, IHS Markit Ltd.

55. Rogers AE, *et al.* (2004) The working hours of hospital staff nurses and patient safety. *Health Affairs (Millwood)*, **23**(4), 202–212.

56. Mueller B, Kinoshita T, Peebles A, Graber MA, Lee S. (2022) Artificial intelligence, and machine learning in emergency medicine: a narrative review. *Acute Medicine & Surgery*, **9**(1), e740.

57. Berlyand Y, Raja AS, Dorner SC *et al.* (2018) How artificial intelligence could transform emergency department operations. *The American Journal of Emergency Medicine*, **36**, 1515–1517.

58. McKinsey Global Institute. (2017) *A future that works: automation, employment, and productivity*. https://www.mckinsey.com/~/media/mckinsey/featured%20insights/Digital%20Disruption/Harnessing%20automation%20for%20a%20future%20that%20works/MGI-A-future-that-works-Executive-summary.ashx

59. GE HealthCare. https://www.gehccommandcenter.com/

60. Modernizing your surgical operations to drive growth for surgeons, healthcare leaders, or leaders. https://qventus.com/

61. ORACLE Cerner. https://www.cerner.com/solutions/command-center

Chapter 19

Why AI is not More Prevalent in Medical Institutions Today?

Introduction

Artificial intelligence (AI) holds great potential to revolutionize healthcare and medicine, offering numerous benefits for patients and healthcare providers. These benefits include early disease detection,[1,2] improvement in diagnostic accuracy[3,4] and the development of personalized diagnostics and therapeutics,[5,6] among others. Indeed, more than 178 AI or machine learning-based medical devices and algorithms have been approved by the U.S. Food and Drug Administration as of October 2022.[7] Yet its prevalence in the medical field remains limited, despite nearly a third of U.S. adults being comfortable with an AI leading their primary care appointment[8] and most physicians having positive attitudes toward the clinical use of AI.[9] This limited uptake can be attributed to the absence of universal approval guidelines, the lack of transparency in algorithmic methods, and the need for collaboration between clinicians and programmers.[10] Overcoming these challenges is crucial to enhance the accuracy and efficiency of medical practices while gaining patient acceptance and trust in algorithmic decision-making. This chapter aims to explore the reasons behind the lack of widespread adoption and utilization of AI in medicine. Understanding these challenges is crucial to unlocking the full potential of AI and maximizing its impact on healthcare delivery and patient outcomes.

Ethical and governance concerns

Ethical considerations in AI implementation

When implementing AI in medicine, ethical considerations must be addressed to ensure the responsible and trustworthy use of these technologies. Two key ethical concerns are patient privacy and data security, as well as bias and fairness in AI algorithms.

Patient privacy and data security are critical aspects that require careful management in AI implementation.[11] The access, use, and control of patient data in the hands of private entities raise concerns regarding privacy and data protection. For example, DeepMind, owned by Google, partnered with Royal Free London NHS in 2016 to use AI for managing patients with acute kidney injury.[12] Critics noted that the patients lacked agency over their data use and privacy impacts were not adequately discussed.[12] A UK health official said patient information was obtained without an appropriate legal basis.[13] Further controversy arose when Google took control of DeepMind's app, effectively transferring UK patient data to the U.S.[14] This shows how private partnerships could annex large quantities of patient data to another jurisdiction — a new risk of big data healthcare AI. The concentration of tech expertise in big companies like Google creates an imbalance where public health institutions can become over-dependent and lose equal standing in partnerships. This makes them more vulnerable to poor privacy protections when implementing commercial healthcare AI products. Safeguarding patient privacy and implementing robust data security measures are essential to maintain trust and protect sensitive health information.[15]

Bias and fairness in AI algorithms pose significant ethical challenges. AI systems learn from historical data, and if that data contains biases, it can perpetuate and amplify them in decision-making processes. Ensuring that AI algorithms are free from bias and produce fair outcomes is decisive in preventing disparities in diagnoses, treatments, and access to care. Therefore, addressing these ethical considerations is paramount to promoting responsible AI implementation in healthcare. By prioritizing patient privacy, data security, and fairness, AI can be harnessed ethically to enhance healthcare delivery and improve patient outcomes.

Regulatory challenges and guidelines

The widespread implementation of AI in hospitals and clinics is limited due to several factors. One major challenge is the absence of universal approval guidelines for regulating AI algorithms in medicine. The FDA regulates some, but not all, AI-enabled products used in healthcare. For the products under its jurisdiction, the FDA plays a vital role in reviewing safety and effectiveness. However, the agency is still evaluating how best to adapt its regulatory approach to AI-enabled medical devices. These devices can evolve rapidly based on new data, sometimes in unpredictable ways. This makes it challenging for the FDA's traditional review framework to keep pace and continuously assess performance. The agency is considering how to update its processes to properly regulate medical AI that changes after approval. This could involve new reporting requirements for AI algorithm changes or periodic reviews. Clear regulatory guidance will be important as innovative AI healthcare products become more prevalent. The FDA is key to developing an oversight framework that ensures patient safety and appropriate use without stifling innovation.[16,17]

Obtaining FDA approval for AI-based trials is further complicated by the need for transparency in scientific methods. Many algorithms rely on intricate mathematics that is often considered a "black box," making it difficult to understand their inner workings. The FDA requires transparency in the algorithm's functionality and decision-making process. However, researchers and companies may be hesitant to expose their valuable proprietary methods and intellectual property, resulting in limited transparency. To address these challenges, it is important to establish comprehensive regulations and guidelines at the international and national levels. Governments around the world are recognizing the need to develop regulations that ensure patient safety, data privacy, and ethical considerations in the use of AI in healthcare. For example, the International Coalition of

Medicines Regulatory Authorities (ICMRA), a global conference of government health bureaucrats, has provided recommendations to help regulators address the challenges posed by AI in global medicines regulation.[18]

Healthcare institutions and organizations also play a role in developing institutional policies and guidelines for the ethical and responsible use of AI in healthcare.[19] These policies ensure that AI technologies are deployed in alignment with the organization's values and objectives. For instance, the Ministry of Health in Singapore has collaborated with relevant authorities to develop the MOH Artificial Intelligence in Healthcare Guidelines (AIHGle), which provide good practices for AI developers and implementers in the healthcare sector.[20] The World Health Organization (WHO) has provided valuable guidance on the ethical and governance aspects of AI in healthcare. Their report titled "Ethics and Governance of Artificial Intelligence for Health"[21] outlines six guiding principles that emphasize the importance of placing ethics and human rights at the core of AI design and implementation. These principles highlight the need for transparency, accountability, inclusiveness, and equity on the use of AI in healthcare.

By establishing international and national regulations, developing institutional policies and guidelines, and adhering to WHO's guiding principles, healthcare professionals can pave the way for the responsible and ethical use of AI in healthcare. Collaboration between regulatory bodies, healthcare institutions, and AI developers is essential to create a supportive environment that ensures patient safety, fosters transparency, and addresses the challenges associated with the implementation of AI in hospitals and clinics.

Technological challenges associated with implementing AI in the healthcare setting

Data availability and quality

One of the primary obstacles to widespread AI development is the limited availability of comprehensive and standardized healthcare data necessary for training them. In this section, we will explore the reasons behind the limited access to diverse and representative datasets in healthcare systems and how it hinders the development and validation of AI models, consequently limiting their effectiveness.

Limited access to comprehensive and standardized healthcare data

Healthcare systems often lack access to comprehensive and standardized data that is vital for training and deploying AI algorithms. The scarcity of high-quality datasets poses a significant challenge to developing accurate and robust AI models in healthcare.[22] Several factors contribute to this issue:

- Fragmented data sources: Healthcare data is often stored in various systems, such as electronic health records (EHRs), imaging databases, and laboratory information systems. These systems may use different data formats, making it challenging to integrate and analyze data from different sources. The lack of standardized formats hampers data interoperability and impedes the development of comprehensive datasets.
- Data privacy and regulatory concerns: The sensitive nature of patient data raises legitimate privacy concerns and necessitates adherence to stringent regulations, such as the Health Insurance Portability and Accountability Act (HIPAA). These regulations protect patient privacy but also impose restrictions on data access, sharing, and usage. Healthcare organizations must navigate complex legal and ethical considerations when accessing and utilizing patient data for AI development.
- Data silos and limited collaboration: Healthcare data is often fragmented across different institutions, creating data silos that hinder collaboration and data sharing. Institutional barriers, concerns about data ownership, and a lack of standardized protocols for data exchange contribute to this challenge. Limited collaboration restricts the availability of diverse datasets necessary for training AI models and inhibits their generalizability.

- Consequences of limited data availability: The limited access to comprehensive and standardized healthcare data has several implications for AI in medicine. Firstly, it restricts the size and diversity of datasets used to train AI models, potentially leading to biased or incomplete representations of patient populations. Additionally, the scarcity of high-quality data hinders the validation and testing of AI algorithms, impeding their accuracy, reliability, and generalizability. Consequently, the adoption of AI in clinical practice is slower than anticipated, as healthcare providers must ensure that the deployed AI models meet rigorous standards of safety, efficacy, and privacy.

Integration with existing healthcare systems

Interoperability issues and lack of standardized data formats

As noted above, healthcare systems often use different data formats and these formats lack interoperability. This makes it very challenging to integrate AI systems seamlessly. Incompatible systems and data formats create barriers to data exchange and interoperability, hampering the integration of AI into existing workflows.

Legacy systems and infrastructure limitations

Many healthcare organizations still rely on legacy systems that are not designed to support AI integration, requiring significant upgrades or replacements. The cost and complexity of upgrading infrastructure pose challenges to implementing AI technologies effectively.

AI algorithm development and validation

Complex algorithms requiring large-scale training and validation

Complex algorithms requiring large-scale training and validation are a significant aspect of AI in medicine. These algorithms are designed to achieve high accuracy and generalizability but require extensive training on large datasets. Moreover, acquiring and labeling such datasets can be resource-intensive and time-consuming. To illustrate this, consider a few examples:

- Cancer diagnosis: In cancer diagnosis, machine learning algorithms are trained on large datasets of medical images, such as mammograms or histopathological slides. These algorithms learn to detect patterns indicative of cancerous cells or tumors. The training process requires access to a large collection of annotated images, which are manually labeled by experts. Obtaining a comprehensive and diverse dataset with accurate annotations is crucial for training robust cancer diagnosis algorithms.
- Deep learning in healthcare: Deep learning algorithms, a subset of AI, have demonstrated remarkable capabilities in various medical applications. For instance, deep neural networks have been employed in speech recognition for acoustic modeling in speech recognition research. These algorithms require extensive training on large datasets of speech recordings to accurately recognize and transcribe spoken words. Training such models involves feeding the algorithm millions of examples of people speaking from scripts, in order to learn the underlying patterns and relationships in speech.
- Predictive models for disease diagnosis: Machine learning techniques are also used to develop predictive models for diagnosing diseases. Researchers have developed models for cancer diagnosis, cardiovascular risk prediction, and other medical conditions. These models require access to large-scale datasets containing patient characteristics, medical history, and clinical outcomes. The algorithms learn from this data to identify relevant patterns and make accurate predictions.

The process of training and validating complex AI algorithms in medicine is resource-intensive due to the need for large, labeled datasets. The availability and quality of these datasets significantly impact the performance and generalizability of the algorithms. Additionally, the challenges of data privacy, regulatory compliance, and data interoperability further complicate the acquisition and utilization of large-scale healthcare datasets for AI training. Nonetheless, efforts are underway to address these challenges and facilitate the development and deployment of AI algorithms in healthcare.

Limited generalizability and transferability of AI models

AI models trained on specific datasets may face challenges in generalizing well to diverse patient populations and different healthcare settings, which can limit their widespread applicability. The performance and generalizability of AI models can be influenced by variations in patient demographics, healthcare practices, and technological infrastructure across different settings.

Cultural and organizational barriers

The successful integration of AI in healthcare is hindered by several cultural and organizational barriers. This section will discuss the key barriers that prevent the full implementation of AI in healthcare facilities and explore the reasons behind them. In most cases, the healthcare sector is known for its traditional and conservative nature, characterized by thorough analysis before implementation and cautious decision-making followed by an incremental process. Traditionally, the medical sector does not integrate technology as quickly as other industries.[23]

Resistance to change

Resistance to change is a common challenge encountered when implementing new technologies, including AI, in healthcare. Healthcare professionals and staff may be resistant to adopting AI due to concerns about disrupting established workflows and practices.

Fear of job displacement

Another significant barrier is the fear of job displacement among healthcare professionals.[24,25] Vinod Khosla, a prominent venture capitalist and Sun Microsystems co-founder, was a keynote speaker at the Health Innovation Summit in 2012. He stated that "AI-machines will replace 80%

of doctors."[26] Statements like Mr. Khosla's, along with the excitement surrounding the human-like capabilities of Chatgpt and MidJourney, suggest to some healthcare professionals that the potential impact of AI on roles and job security could be devastating. This raises a lot of concern and anxiety among healthcare professionals. For example, a study by Reeder and Lee, from the Journal Clinical Imaging (2022), showed that awareness of AI's image analysis capabilities significantly lowered student's preference for choosing radiology as a career.[27] Additional research and studies should be incorporated to explore the fear of job displacement across various healthcare professions and specialties.

Fear of professional deskilling

Healthcare professionals worry that as AI systems take over certain tasks, there may be a risk of deskilling, where their expertise and decision-making abilities may be diminished.[28] This concern is understandable as the use of AI in areas such as diagnosis prediction and treatment recommendation, the core skills for most physicians, become more accurate and more prevalent.[30] As AI technology continues to advance, it is important to address the concerns of healthcare professionals through education, training, and ongoing collaboration to ensure the successful and responsible integration of AI into clinical practice.

Lack of awareness and understanding

The successful integration of AI relies on the knowledge and acceptance by healthcare professionals. A lack of awareness and understanding of AI technology and its capabilities can hinder its adoption. Research findings and surveys should be included to demonstrate the current level of awareness and understanding of AI among healthcare professionals, highlighting the need for educational initiatives and training programs.

Limited funding and resource allocation

The financial challenges associated with implementing AI technologies pose a significant barrier to their widespread adoption. Limited funding and resource allocation can impede the progress and integration of AI in healthcare systems.

Cost implications

Integrating AI into healthcare systems requires substantial investments in infrastructure, software development, data storage, and computational resources. These costs can be prohibitive for healthcare organizations, especially those with limited financial resources. Allocating funds for AI projects may compete with other healthcare priorities, making it challenging to secure sufficient resources for AI implementation.

Resource constraints

Limited funding restricts the ability of healthcare organizations to allocate resources effectively. With competing priorities, AI projects may not receive the necessary financial support, leading to delays and reduced progress in adopting AI technologies. Smaller hospitals or those in low-resource settings may face even greater resource constraints, exacerbating existing healthcare disparities.

Training and education

Effective implementation of AI in healthcare requires specialized skills and knowledge. However, training healthcare professionals and staff members to effectively use and interpret AI-powered tools can be resource-intensive. Limited funding may restrict the availability of training programs and educational resources, in turn, hindering the ability of the workforce to leverage AI effectively.

Infrastructure and data challenges

AI algorithms rely on large amounts of high-quality data for training and validation. Collecting, storing, and managing the necessary data is expensive and may be inaccessible for institutions with limited resources.

Insufficient infrastructure and outdated data systems can impede the implementation of AI solutions.

Misaligned incentives

The concept of misaligned incentives is an important consideration when discussing the widespread adoption of AI in healthcare. While innovations in algorithmic transparency, data collection, and regulation are crucial for successful AI implementation, another vital aspect deserving equal attention is the role of decision-makers in the healthcare sector. The assumption is often made that resolving issues related to algorithms, data availability, and regulations will lead to accelerated AI adoption, benefiting society. However, the ultimate decision to adopt AI technology lies with healthcare decision-makers. These decision-makers, who are often medical professionals, may feel threatened by AI algorithms that could potentially replace them, or at least some tasks they currently perform.

In a Brookings Institute study in March 2022,[29] researchers explored AI adoption rates through an analysis of AI-related job postings in healthcare. They found that adoption rates vary depending on the type of job and the hospital management structure. AI skills were more likely to be listed in administrative or research roles than in clinical roles. Hospitals with an integrated salary model, typically led by individuals with management expertise, demonstrated a higher adoption rate of AI for administrative and clinical roles but not for research roles, compared to hospitals more likely to be managed by doctors. Interestingly, teaching hospitals showed no significant difference in their adoption rate compared to other hospitals. One possible interpretation of these patterns is that hospitals with an integrated salary model, led by professional managers, recognize the potential benefits of AI in clinical and administrative settings. In contrast, hospitals led by doctors may have different priorities or concerns, leading to slower AI adoption. However, it is crucial to consider that there are various reasons that may contribute to the slow adoption of AI in hospitals beyond the management structure. Doctor-led hospitals may be more aware of other adoption challenges, such as algorithmic limitations, data access constraints, and regulatory hurdles, which require careful consideration before implementing AI technologies.

Economic considerations in implementing AI in healthcare

Implementing AI in healthcare requires careful consideration of the associated financial implications. The cost of AI implementation and infrastructure is a significant factor that needs to be addressed. It involves a substantial initial investment for acquiring AI technologies and establishing the necessary infrastructure, including the purchase of AI systems, hardware and software upgrades, and the implementation of robust data security measures. Additionally, ongoing expenses such as software updates, system monitoring, and staff training contribute to the overall costs of AI implementation.

To justify these expenses, healthcare organizations often conduct cost-effectiveness analyses and evaluate the return on investment (ROI) associated with AI implementation. It is imperative to assess the potential benefits that AI systems can bring, such as improved efficiency, enhanced diagnostic accuracy, and better patient outcomes. By carefully evaluating these benefits, healthcare organizations can determine the long-term value and financial viability of implementing AI in their operations.

Integrating AI into existing reimbursement and payment models presents challenges in the healthcare industry. One of the key challenges is defining appropriate reimbursement codes and pricing models for AI-based services. The dynamic nature of AI technologies, which continually evolve, makes it difficult to establish standardized pricing structures that accurately reflect the value of AI services. Additionally, aligning AI reimbursement with existing healthcare financing systems is a complex task. Healthcare providers and payers must navigate through regulatory frameworks and negotiate agreements that appropriately capture the value and impact of AI technologies. This alignment is essential to ensure fair reimbursement for AI services while maintaining the financial sustainability of healthcare organizations.

To address these challenges, a reimbursement framework that involves multiple stakeholders is recommended. The framework should include the participation of patients, policymakers, clinicians, regulators, provider organizations, bioethicists, and AI creators. By engaging these stakeholders, it is possible to develop a comprehensive and sustainable reimbursement model for AI in healthcare. This framework should consider ethics, workflow, cost, and value, and should be based on a collaborative approach that ensures quality of care, healthcare equity, mitigation of potential bias, and improved clinical outcomes for patients and populations.

Implementing AI in healthcare requires careful consideration of the economic aspects. The cost of AI implementation and infrastructure, along with the challenges associated with reimbursement and payment models, need to be addressed. Through rigorous cost-effectiveness analyses, ROI evaluations, and the involvement of various stakeholders, healthcare organizations can determine the long-term value and financial viability of AI systems. By aligning reimbursement with existing healthcare financing systems, fair reimbursement for AI services can be achieved while ensuring the financial sustainability of healthcare organizations. It is essential to develop a reimbursement framework that considers the dynamic nature of AI technologies and actively involves all stakeholders to realize the full potential of AI in improving healthcare outcomes.

Future directions and potential solutions for the adoption of AI systems in healthcare institutions

The adoption of AI systems in healthcare institutions still faces challenges despite its potential to revolutionize patient care and outcomes. This section explores future directions and potential solutions to overcome these challenges and promote the wider implementation of AI in healthcare. Key areas of focus include addressing barriers to adoption, ensuring regulatory compliance, promoting collaboration and partnerships, enhancing data infrastructure, and fostering trust and acceptance among healthcare professionals and patients.

Addressing barriers to adoption

- Digitalization and infrastructure: The healthcare sector lags in digitalization, which hinders the implementation of AI systems. Efforts should be made to improve digital infrastructure, including EHRs, data interoperability, and secure data sharing.

- Funding models: Current funding models in healthcare systems often prioritize traditional hardware and drugs, making it challenging to allocate resources for AI solutions. Governments and healthcare organizations should explore innovative funding mechanisms to support the development and implementation of AI technologies in healthcare.

Ensuring regulatory compliance

- Ethical and legal frameworks: The development of comprehensive ethical and legal frameworks is crucial to address concerns regarding patient privacy, data security, and liability in AI-driven healthcare. Regulatory bodies should work closely with stakeholders to establish guidelines that govern the responsible and ethical use of AI in healthcare.
- Standards and certification: Establishing standards and certification processes for AI systems in healthcare can ensure their safety, effectiveness, and interoperability. Collaboration between regulatory bodies, industry leaders, and research institutions can contribute to the development of these standards.

Promoting collaboration and partnerships

- Public-private collaboration: Collaboration between healthcare institutions, technology companies, and government agencies can accelerate the adoption of AI in healthcare. Public-private partnerships can provide the necessary resources, expertise, and funding to overcome implementation challenges and facilitate knowledge sharing.
- Interdisciplinary collaboration: Encouraging collaboration among healthcare professionals, data scientists, engineers, and researchers can foster innovation and drive the implementation of AI systems in healthcare. Interdisciplinary research projects, conferences, and forums can facilitate knowledge exchange and promote a holistic approach to AI implementation.

Enhancing data infrastructure

- Data accessibility and quality: Improvements in data availability, accessibility, and quality are crucial for the successful implementation of AI systems in healthcare. Efforts should focus on data standardization, data governance, and the development of secure data-sharing platforms.

- Data integration and interoperability: AI systems can benefit by using integrated data obtained from various sources, including EHRs, medical imaging, and wearable devices. Establishing interoperability standards and technologies can facilitate the seamless integration and analysis of diverse datasets for AI-driven applications.

Fostering trust and acceptance

- Explainable and interpretable AI: AI algorithms should be designed to provide clear explanations and justifications for their decisions. Developing explainable AI models can enhance transparency, facilitate trust-building, and encourage acceptance among healthcare professionals and patients.
- Education and training: Investing in AI education and training programs for healthcare professionals is essential. Integrating AI education into medical curricula and providing continuous professional development opportunities can empower healthcare professionals to understand, evaluate, and effectively use AI-powered tools.

The adoption of AI systems in healthcare institutions can be facilitated by addressing barriers to adoption, ensuring regulatory compliance, promoting collaboration and partnerships, enhancing data infrastructure, and fostering trust and acceptance. By focusing on these future directions and implementing potential solutions, healthcare institutions can harness the full potential of AI to improve patient care, enhance outcomes, and transform the healthcare landscape.

Conclusion

The adoption of AI systems in healthcare institutions holds great potential for revolutionizing patient care and outcomes. However, several challenges need to be addressed to promote wider implementation. Future directions and potential solutions include: 1) Efforts to improve digital infrastructure, such as EHRs, data interoperability, and secure data sharing, are critical to overcoming barriers to adoption. Healthcare organizations and governments should explore innovative funding mechanisms to allocate resources for AI solutions in healthcare. 2) Comprehensive ethical and legal frameworks are needed to address concerns regarding patient privacy, data security, and liability. Regulatory bodies should collaborate with stakeholders to establish guidelines that govern the responsible and ethical use of AI in healthcare. Additionally, establishing standards and certification processes can ensure the safety, effectiveness, and interoperability of AI systems in healthcare. 3) Promoting collaboration and partnerships is essential for accelerating the adoption of AI in healthcare. Public-private collaborations can provide resources, expertise, and funding to overcome implementation challenges and facilitate knowledge sharing. Interdisciplinary collaboration among healthcare professionals, data scientists, engineers, and researchers can foster innovation and drive AI implementation. 4) Enhancing data infrastructure involves improving data accessibility, quality, and interoperability. Standardization, data governance, and the development of secure data-sharing platforms are necessary to enable successful AI implementation in healthcare. 5) Fostering trust and acceptance among healthcare professionals and patients can be achieved through the development of explainable and interpretable AI models. Clear explanations and justifications for AI algorithms' decisions enhance transparency and build trust. Investing in AI education and training programs for healthcare professionals is also crucial to empower them to effectively use AI-powered tools.

By addressing these future directions and implementing potential solutions, healthcare institutions can harness the full potential of AI to improve patient care, enhance outcomes, and transform the healthcare landscape. Collaborative efforts between stakeholders, robust regulatory frameworks, and investments in digital infrastructure and education play crucial roles in overcoming the challenges and facilitating the wider adoption of AI in healthcare.

References

1. Kerut EK, To F, Summers KL, Sheahan C, Sheahan M. (2019) Statistical and machine learning methodology for abdominal aortic aneurysm prediction from ultrasound screenings. *Echocardiography*, **36**, 1989–1996.
2. Le S, Hoffman J, *et al.* (2019) Pediatric severe sepsis prediction using machine learning. *Frontiers in Pediatrics*, **7**, 413.
3. Erickson BJ, Korfiatis P, *et al.* (2017) Machine learning for medical imaging. *RadioGraphics*, **37**, 505–515.
4. Serag A, Ion-Margineanu A, Qureshi H, *et al.* (2019) Translational AI and deep learning in diagnostic pathology. *Frontiers in Medicine (Lausanne)*, **6**, 185.
5. Mo X, Chen X, Li H, Li J, *et al.* (2019) Early and accurate prediction of clinical response to methotrexate treatment in juvenile idiopathic arthritis using machine learning. *Frontiers in Pharmacology*, **10**, 1155.
6. Ghosh R, Warier P, Vaccaro B, *et al.* (2018) Machine learning methods improve prognostication, identify clinically distinct phenotypes, and detect heterogeneity in response to therapy in a large cohort of heart failure patients. *Journal of the American Heart Association*, **7**, e008081.
7. FDA. Artificial Intelligence and Machine Learning (Ai/Ml)-Enabled Medical Devices. (2021) https://www.fda.gov/medical-devices/software-medical-device-samd/artificial-intelligence-and-machine-learning-aiml-enabled-medical-devices?utm_source=FDALinkedin#resources
8. Padgett Z. Outbreaks near me|SurveyMonkey poll: AI isn't disrupting healthcare — yet. https://www.surveymonkey.com/curiosity/ai-isnt-disrupting-healthcare-yet/
9. Chen M, Zhang B, Cai Z, Seery S, Gonzalez MJ, Ali NM, Ren R, Qiao Y, Xue P, Jiang Y. (2022) Acceptance of clinical artificial intelligence among physicians and medical students: a systematic review with cross-sectional survey. *Frontiers in Medicine (Lausanne)*, 9, 990604.
10. He J, Baxter SL, Xu J, Xu J, Zhou X, Zhang K. (2019) The practical implementation of artificial intelligence technologies in medicine. *Nature Medicine*, **25**, 30–36.
11. Murdoch B. (2021) Privacy and artificial intelligence: challenges for protecting health information in a new era. *BMC Medical Ethics*, **22**, 122.

12. Cuttler M. (2019) Transforming health care: how artificial intelligence is reshaping the medical landscape. https://www.cbc.ca/news/health/artificial-intelligence-health-care-1.5110892
13. Iacobucci G. (2017) Patient data were shared with Google on an "inappropriate legal basis", says NHS data guardian. *The BMJ*, **357**, j2439.
14. Vincent J. (2018) Privacy advocates sound the alarm after Google grabs DeepMind UK health app. https://www.theverge.com/2018/11/14/18094874/google-deepmind-health-app-privacy-concerns-uk-nhs-medical-data
15. Baowaly MK, Lin CC, Liu CL, Chen KT. (2019) Synthesizing electronic health records using improved generative adversarial networks. *Journal of the American Medical Informatics Association*, **26**(3), 228–241.
16. U.S. Food and Drug Administration. (2021) Artificial Intelligence/Machine Learning (AI/ML)-Based Software as a Medical Device (SaMD) Action Plan. https://www.fda.gov/media/145022/download
17. U.S. Food and Drug Administration. (2019) Proposed Regulatory Framework for Modifications to Artificial Intelligence/Machine Learning (AI/ML)-Based Software as a Medical Device (SaMD) — Discussion Paper and Request for Feedback. https://www.fda.gov/media/122535/download
18. International Coalition of Medicines Regulatory Authorities (ICMRA). https://www.ema.europa.eu/en/partners-networks/international-activities/multilateral-coalitions-initiatives/international-coalition-medicines-regulatory-authorities-icmra
19. Siala H, Wang Y. (2022) SHIFTing artificial intelligence to be responsible in healthcare: A systematic review. *Social Science & Medicine (1982)*, **296**, 114782.
20. MOH's artificial intelligence in healthcare guidelines (AIHGle). https://form.gov.sg/5e43a4328a8e1700110d5af3
21. WHO guidance. (2021) Ethics and governance of artificial intelligence for health. https://www.who.int/publications/i/item/9789240029200
22. Hulsen T. (2020) Sharing is caring — data sharing initiatives in healthcare. *International Journal of Environmental Research and Public Health*, **17**, 3046.
23. Hermes S, Riasanow T, Clemons EK, Böhm M, Krcmar H. (2020) The digital transformation of the healthcare industry: exploring the rise of emerging platform ecosystems and their influence on the role of patients. *Journal of Business Research*, **13**(3), 1033–1069.
24. Doraiswamy PM, Blease C, Bodner K. (2020) Artificial intelligence and the future of psychiatry: insights from a global physician survey. *Artificial Intelligence in Medicine*, **102**, 101753.

25. Sarwar S, Dent A, Faust K, Richer M, Djuric U, Van Ommeren R, *et al.* (2019) Physician perspectives on integration of artificial intelligence into diagnostic pathology. *npj Digital Medicine*, **2**(1), 1–7.
26. Farr C. (2017) Here's why one tech investor thinks some doctors will be 'obsolete' in five years. https://www.yahoo.com/news/heres-why-one-tech-investor-182821068.html
27. Kristen Reeder, Hwan Lee. (2022) Impact of artificial intelligence on US medical students' choice of radiology. *Clinical Imaging*, **81**, 67–71.
28. Aquino YSJ, *et al.* (2023) Utopia versus dystopia: professional perspectives on the impact of healthcare artificial intelligence on clinical roles and skills. *International Journal of Medical Informatics*, **169**, 104903.
29. Goldfarb A, Teodoridis F. (2022) Why is AI adoption in health care lagging. https://www.brookings.edu/articles/why-is-ai-adoption-in-health-care-lagging/
30. Eriksen AV, Möller S, Ryg J. (2023) Use of GPT-4 to diagnose complex clinical cases. *NEJM AI*, **1**(1), AIp2300031.

Index

www.ingramcontent.com/pod-product-compliance
Lightning Source LLC
Chambersburg PA
CBHW061621220326
41598CB00026BA/3842